# The
# EASY
# ADULT
# ACTIVITY
# BOOK

## Includes Easy Picture Puzzles, Coloring Pages, and Word Searches

### By Joy  Kinnest

Lomic Books

# The
# EASY ADULT ACTIVITY BOOK

\*\*\*

## By Joy Kinnest

\*\*\*

## ISBN: 978-1-988923-23-9

Published by Lomic Books
Kitchener, Ontario

\*\*\*

\*\*\*

## Disclaimer

The author and publisher have worked hard to make sure that the puzzles
and the solutions in this book are accurate; however, the reader should
be aware that errors and omissions may occur. The author and publisher
disclaim any liability to any person or party for any loss resulting from
reliance on any information in this book.

\*\*\*

## For More Puzzles & Activity Books

Lomic Books publishes many high quality puzzle books
and adult activity books. For more on these books please check out:

### www.LomicBooks.com

# CONTENTS

Introduction, Page 4

# INTRODUCTION

Welcome to *The Easy Adult Activity Book!*

This activity book is filled with lots of fun activities including easy picture puzzles, word searches and coloring pages.

To make this activity book easy to use, you will find:

- Large print and clear images are used throughout this book.

- Each easy, relaxing coloring page has a light gray quotation on the back of the page, to protect your artwork on the other side.

- At the beginning of each puzzle section, you will find solving tips for each activity!

We hope you have a terrific time doing the activities in this book.

Enjoy!

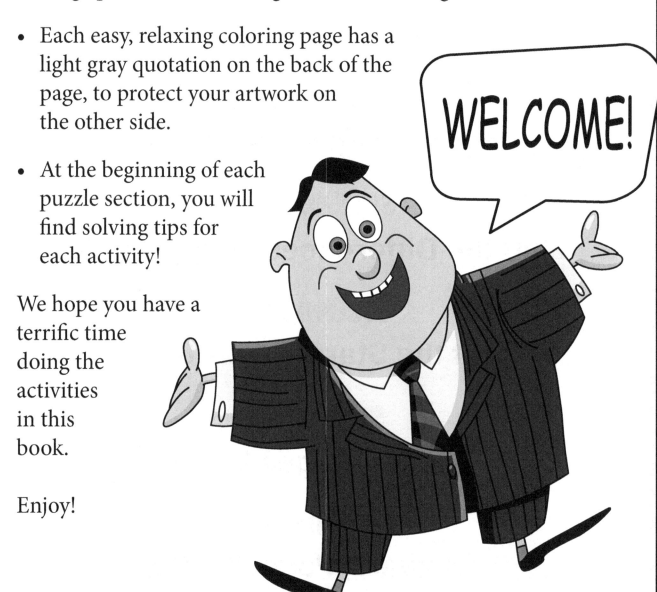

WELCOME!

# SPOT THE ODD ONE OUT

This section is full of 'Spot the Odd One Out' puzzles. The goal for each puzzle is to find the picture that is different from the rest.

## An Example

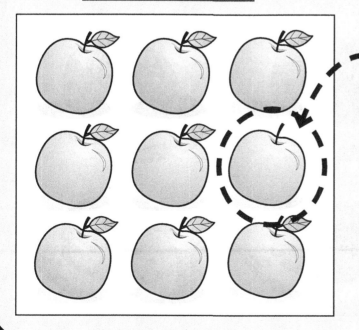

This apple is different. It is missing a leaf.

HINT: There is only one picture that is different.

# FIND THE HAT THAT IS DIFFERENT FROM THE REST

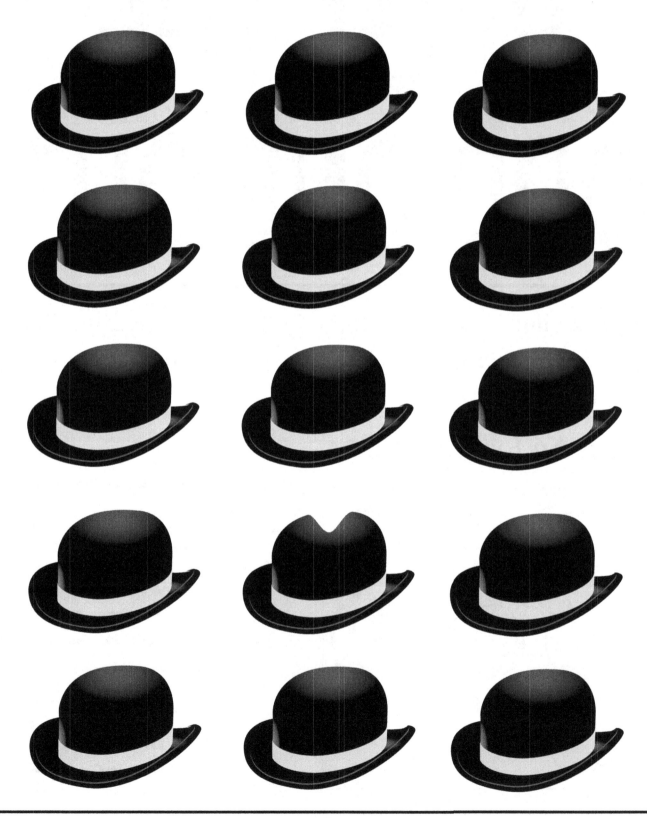

# FIND THE PANDA THAT IS DIFFERENT FROM THE REST

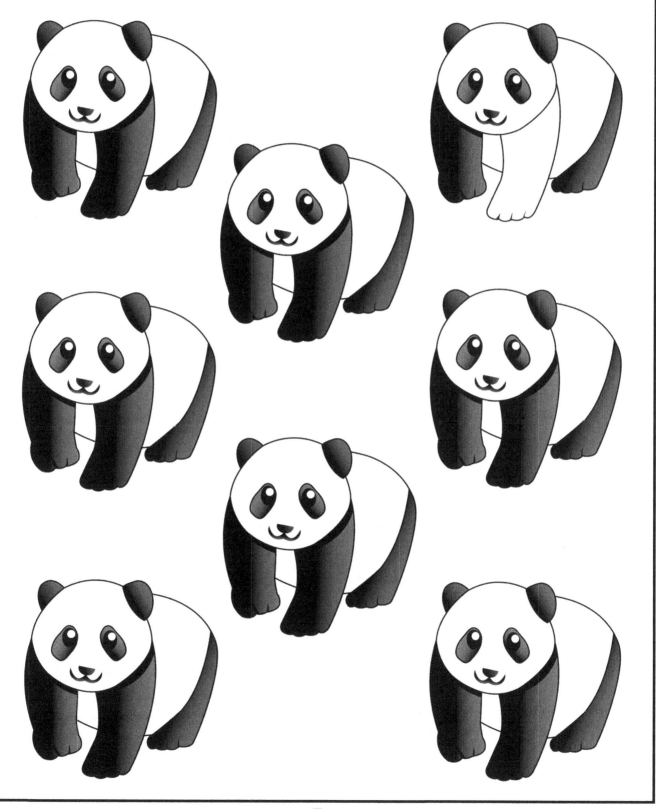

# FIND THE FLOWER THAT IS DIFFERENT FROM THE REST

# FIND THE LADY THAT IS
# DIFFERENT FROM THE REST

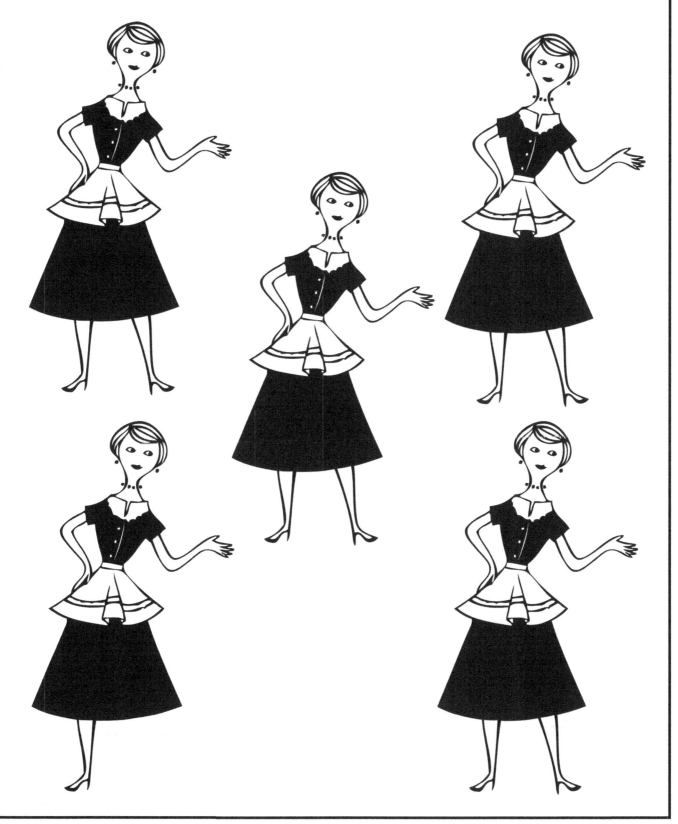

# FIND THE DRINK THAT IS DIFFERENT FROM THE REST

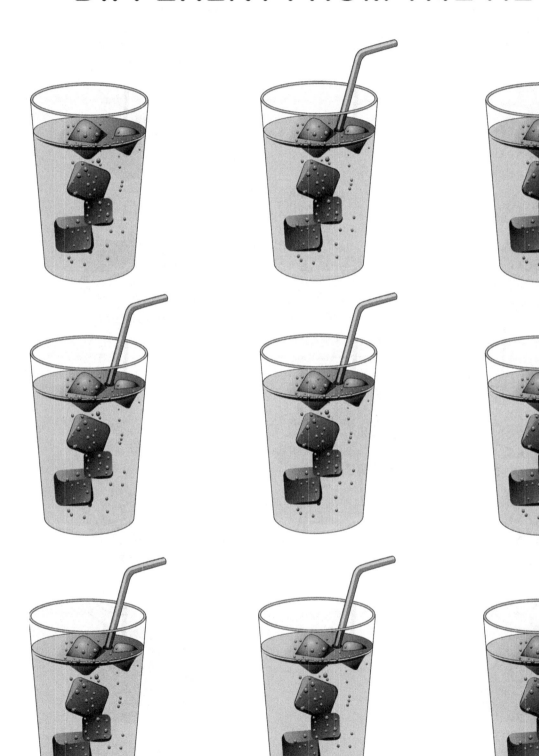

# FIND THE NOTEBOOK THAT IS DIFFERENT FROM THE REST

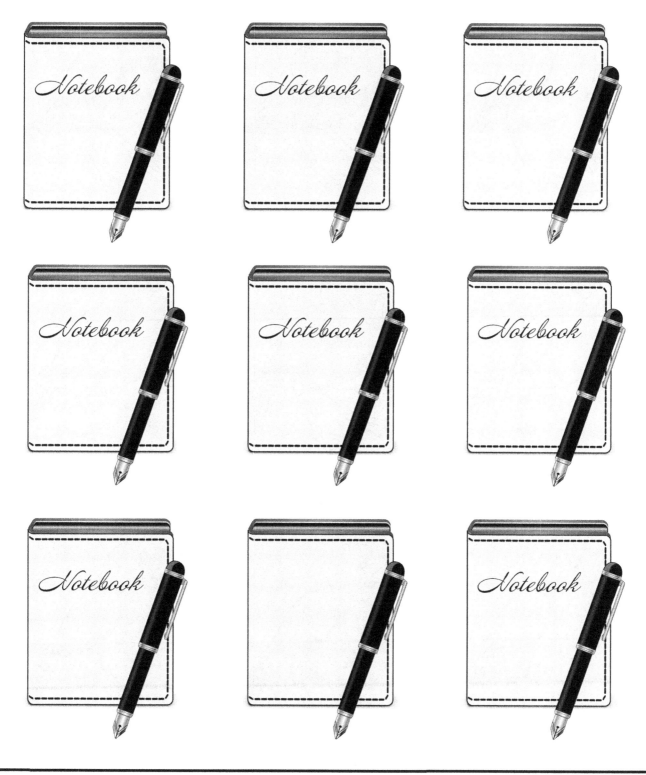

# FIND THE BIRD THAT IS DIFFERENT FROM THE REST

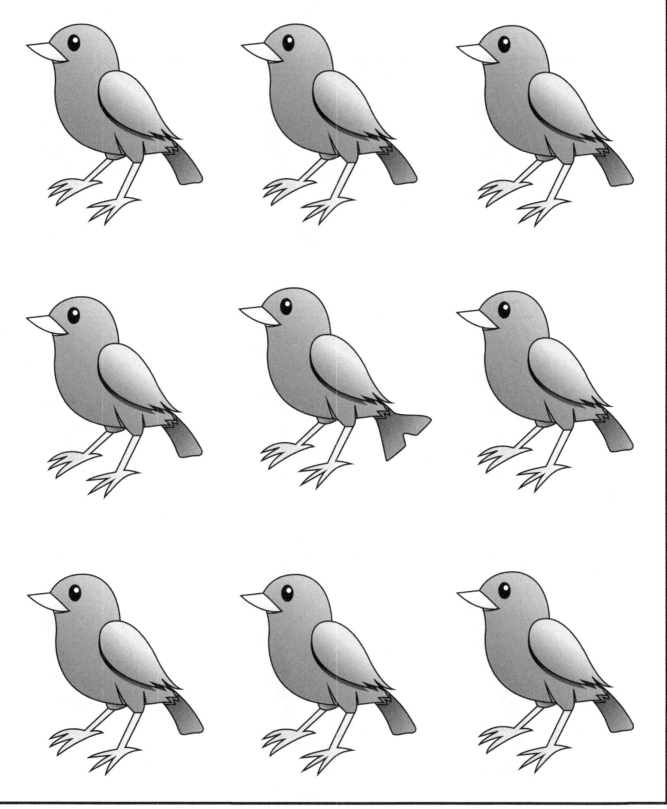

# FIND THE BAG OF SEEDS THAT IS DIFFERENT FROM THE REST

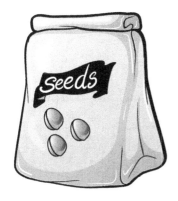 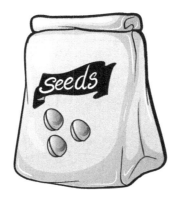 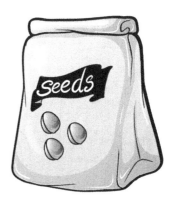

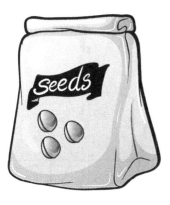 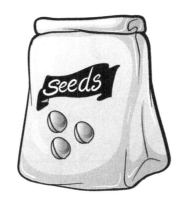 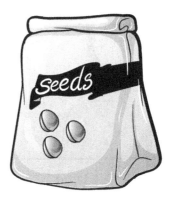

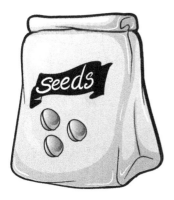 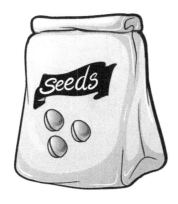 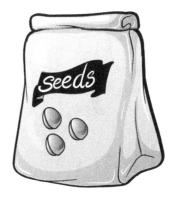

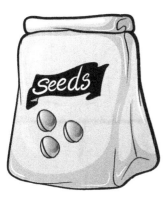 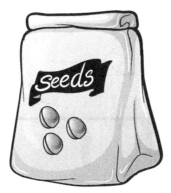 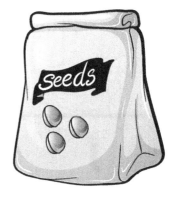

# FIND THE CHAIR THAT IS DIFFERENT FROM THE REST

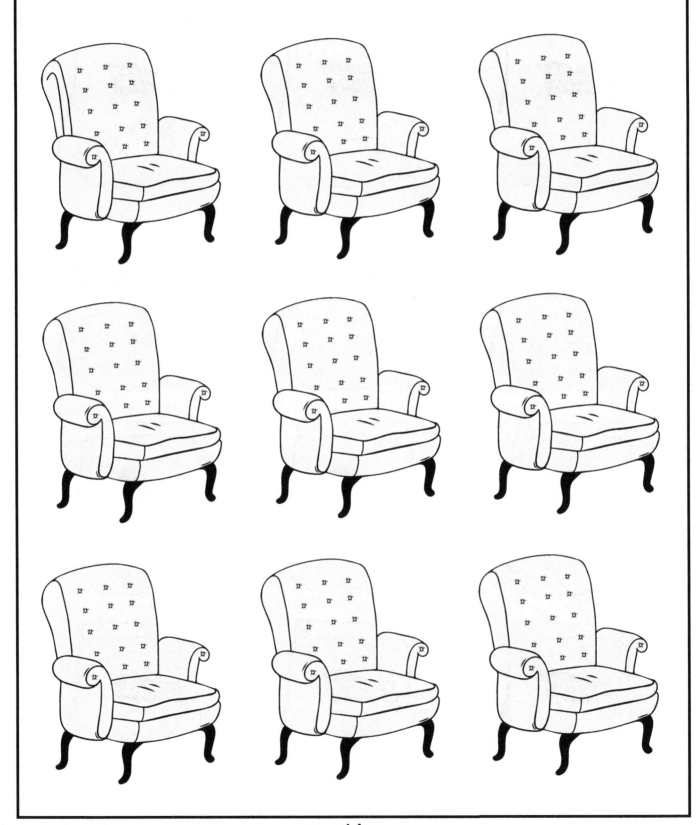

# FIND THE LAMP THAT IS DIFFERENT FROM THE REST

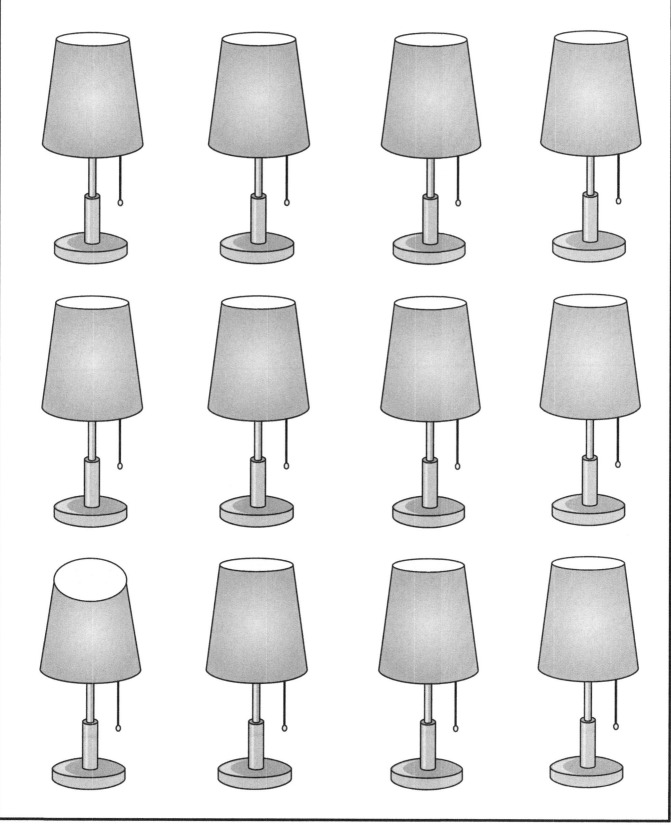

# FIND THE RABBIT THAT IS DIFFERENT FROM THE REST

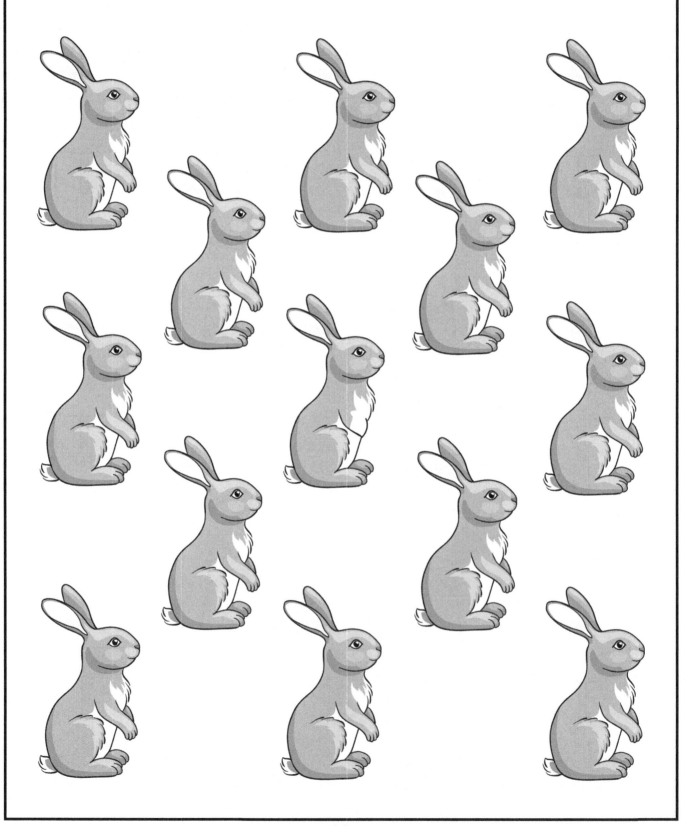

# FIND THE FOX THAT IS DIFFERENT FROM THE REST

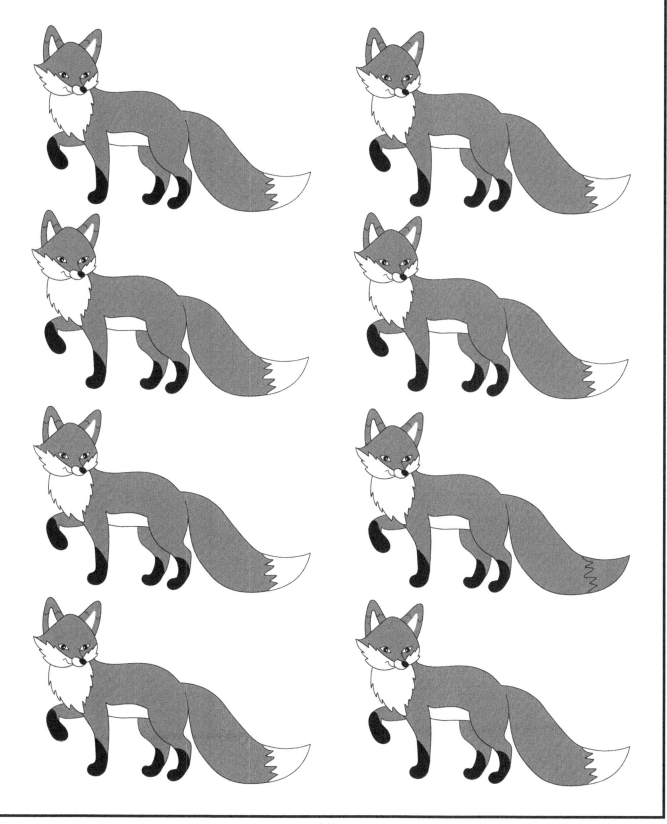

# FIND THE BANANA THAT IS DIFFERENT FROM THE REST

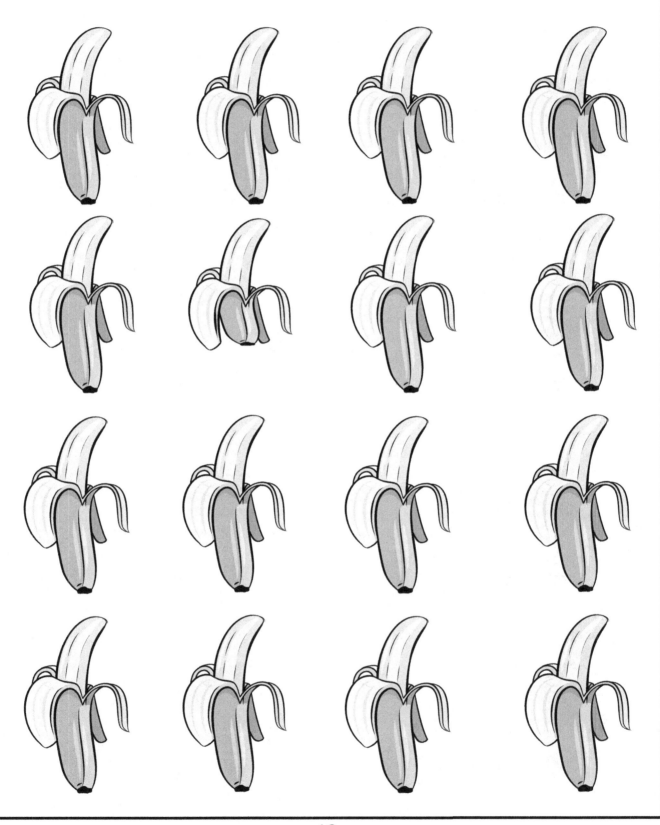

# FIND THE CHOCOLATE BAR THAT IS DIFFERENT FROM THE REST

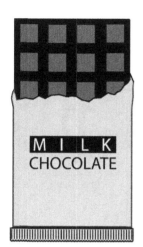 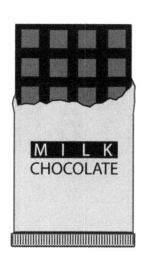 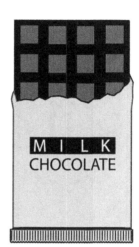 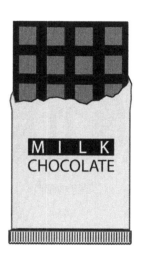

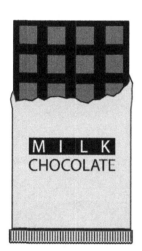 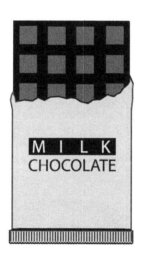 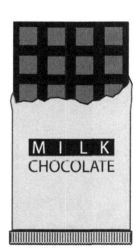 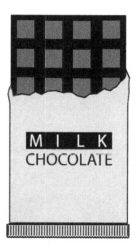

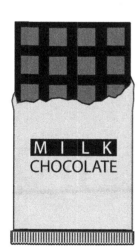 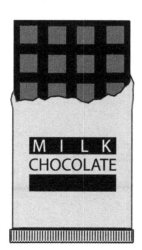 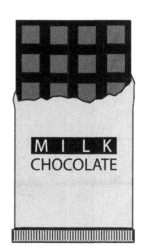 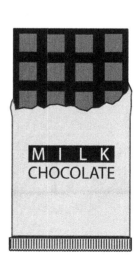

# FIND THE BILLIARD BALL THAT IS DIFFERENT FROM THE REST

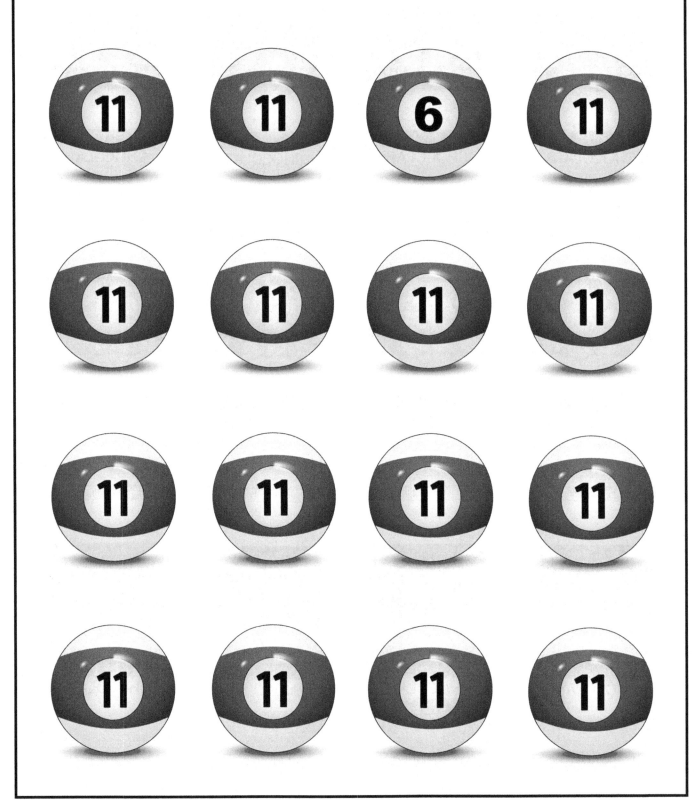

# WORD SEARCHES

This section is full of 'Word Search' puzzles. The goal is to find words in the square. Words are located only in an across or down direction.

## An Example

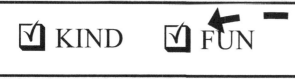

☑ KIND    ☑ FUN

Check the box when you find the word.

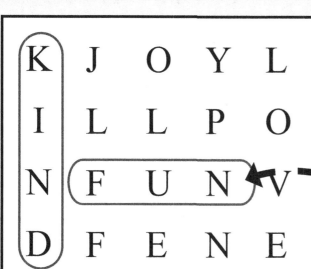

| K | J | O | Y | L |
| I | L | L | P | O |
| N | F | U | N | V |
| D | F | E | N | E |

Circle the word when you find it in the square!

# RADIO

Find the words listed below in the square. If you want, check off the words as you find them.

## WORD LIST:

☐ MUSIC ☐ TRACK ☐ LIVE

☐ TALK ☐ SHOW ☐ HOST

☐ RECORD ☐ LISTEN ☐ FORMAT

| | | | | | | | | | |
|---|---|---|---|---|---|---|---|---|---|
| H | O | S | T | M | L | I | V | E | W |
| T | R | A | C | K | G | L | N | O | U |
| W | Q | F | E | T | R | I | G | M | F |
| V | F | V | A | A | Q | S | H | L | O |
| R | E | C | O | R | D | T | X | T | R |
| P | S | H | D | G | R | E | Y | A | M |
| H | T | S | H | O | W | N | F | L | A |
| M | U | S | I | C | T | F | U | K | T |

# FARM

Find the words listed below in the square. If you want, check off the words as you find them.

## WORD LIST:

☐ BARN     ☐ FENCE     ☐ CROP

☐ GROW     ☐ EGGS     ☐ PIG

☐ GOAT     ☐ TRACTOR     ☐ SHOVEL

```
B Y E O F E N C E D
A K T V G Z V H G H
R V S P R U G X O E
N W L G R O W Z A G
S K T E J B W S T G
T R A C T O R P O S
F S H O V E L I D Y
C R O P P P V N G O K
```

# CARDS

Find the words listed below in the square. If you want, check off the words as you find them.

## WORD LIST:

☐ EUCHRE      ☐ BRIDGE      ☐ UNO

☐ SPEED       ☐ POKER       ☐ WAR

☐ HEARTS      ☐ SPADES      ☐ RUMMY

```
E  W  F  P  O  K  E  R  B  H
U  S  P  A  D  E  S  B  V  E
C  Y  P  G  E  X  S  X  W  A
H  K  Z  L  S  V  P  R  A  R
R  I  O  R  T  M  E  O  R  T
E  E  Q  W  W  E  E  S  Y  S
B  R  I  D  G  E  D  E  H  V
R  U  M  M  Y  J  U  N  O  C
```

# — HAPPY —

Find the words listed below in the square. If you want, check off the words as you find them.

## WORD LIST:

- ☐ CHEER
- ☐ SMILE
- ☐ BLISS
- ☐ JOYFUL
- ☐ GRATEFUL
- ☐ MOOD
- ☐ GLAD
- ☐ MERRY
- ☐ JOLLY

| J | M | C | H | E | E | R | U | S | M |
|---|---|---|---|---|---|---|---|---|---|
| O | K | M | D | E | E | H | B | M | E |
| Y | M | P | R | P | J | S | L | I | R |
| F | J | O | L | L | Y | M | I | L | R |
| U | Q | T | J | Q | F | I | S | E | Y |
| L | D | X | A | Z | Z | Q | S | W | M |
| M | O | O | D | X | G | L | A | D | C |
| H | G | R | A | T | E | F | U | L | V |

# — VEGETABLES —

Find the words listed below in the square. If you want, check off the words as you find them.

## WORD LIST:

☐ LETTUCE     ☐ SPINACH     ☐ RADISH

☐ CARROT     ☐ TURNIP     ☐ POTATO

☐ KALE     ☐ CELERY     ☐ LEEK

```
T U R N I P L A M L
C E L E R Y E A S E
W P S K H J T P P E
H P Z L Q H T O I K
C A R R O T U T N L
G W Q O L C C A A R
R A D I S H E T C I
K A L E Q B Q O H U
```

# — THAT'S FUNNY —

Find the words listed below in the square. If you want, check off the words as you find them.

## WORD LIST:

- ☐ COMEDY
- ☐ LAUGH
- ☐ SILLY
- ☐ RIDDLE
- ☐ JOKE
- ☐ TONE
- ☐ QUIRKY
- ☐ SKIT
- ☐ HUMOR

| C | A | R | Z | E | S | G | J | T | S |
|---|---|---|---|---|---|---|---|---|---|
| O | S | K | I | T | T | K | O | O | I |
| M | G | X | M | G | Q | N | K | N | L |
| E | R | I | D | D | L | E | E | E | L |
| D | H | B | N | C | G | X | M | I | Y |
| Y | H | U | M | O | R | T | S | P | E |
| L | S | Y | Q | U | I | R | K | Y | S |
| L | A | U | G | H | Y | F | X | C | H |

# — BEDROOM —

Find the words listed below in the square. If you want, check off the words as you find them.

## WORD LIST:

❑ CLOSET  ❑ WINDOW  ❑ CLOCK

❑ SHELF  ❑ LAMP  ❑ BLANKET

❑ PILLOW  ❑ RUG  ❑ BED

| | | | | | | | | | |
|---|---|---|---|---|---|---|---|---|---|
| S | S | S | C | B | E | D | C | P | V |
| H | U | C | L | J | C | W | X | I | B |
| E | I | R | O | V | B | S | S | L | L |
| L | D | E | C | V | F | J | D | L | A |
| F | C | M | K | N | D | X | R | O | N |
| E | W | I | N | D | O | W | U | W | K |
| C | L | O | S | E | T | I | G | F | E |
| F | J | F | L | L | A | M | P | L | T |

# — TELEPHONE —

Find the words listed below in the square. If you want, check off the words as you find them.

## WORD LIST:

☐ NUMBER ☐ CHAT ☐ CALL

☐ HOLD ☐ ANSWER ☐ TALK

☐ DIAL ☐ MESSAGE ☐ RING

| R | C | A | L | L | U | M | U | V | T |
|---|---|---|---|---|---|---|---|---|---|
| I | U | N | G | Q | V | E | I | D | A |
| N | Y | M | H | S | E | S | V | C | L |
| G | K | I | A | V | N | S | U | H | K |
| H | O | L | D | W | V | A | J | A | X |
| A | N | S | W | E | R | G | U | T | O |
| S | D | I | A | L | I | E | N | B | Q |
| N | U | M | B | E | R | O | H | F | H |

# — HAIR CUT —

Find the words listed below in the square. If you want, check off the words as you find them.

## WORD LIST:

☐ COMB          ☐ SCISSORS          ☐ BRUSH

☐ TRIM          ☐ SPRAY             ☐ DYE

☐ STYLIST       ☐ GEL               ☐ WASH

```
L  W  A  S  H  J  T  A  D  B
S  C  I  S  S  O  R  S  Y  R
C  O  M  B  Y  P  G  E  E  U
I  R  O  T  A  M  Y  B  Y  S
O  X  F  W  C  O  B  R  V  H
S  P  R  A  Y  Y  C  D  G  H
S  T  Y  L  I  S  T  L  E  D
S  L  N  T  R  I  M  O  L  B
```

# PETS

Find the words listed below in the square. If you want, check off the words as you find them.

## WORD LIST:

- ☐ DOG
- ☐ BIRD
- ☐ FISH
- ☐ TURTLE
- ☐ HAMSTER
- ☐ GERBIL
- ☐ CAT
- ☐ RABBIT
- ☐ MOUSE

```
F  B  I  R  D  X  D  Y  H  E
I  P  M  X  C  N  M  I  A  Y
S  C  Z  D  A  N  E  R  M  Y
H  U  I  A  T  Q  W  A  S  L
M  O  U  S  E  Y  M  B  T  X
X  T  U  R  T  L  E  B  E  D
K  N  A  X  U  S  A  I  R  O
G  E  R  B  I  L  R  T  A  G
```

# — KITCHEN —

Find the words listed below in the square. If you want, check off the words as you find them.

## WORD LIST:

☐ FRIDGE          ☐ SINK          ☐ KNIFE

☐ BOWL           ☐ STOVE        ☐ PLATE

☐ FORK           ☐ TABLE        ☐ SPOON

```
S  I  N  K  I  T  F  P  K  P
F  R  I  D  G  E  O  H  N  L
S  M  E  X  U  N  R  T  I  A
S  P  O  O  N  T  K  H  F  T
L  U  L  E  I  M  O  L  E  E
O  G  X  B  O  W  L  X  A  K
I  X  S  N  S  T  O  V  E  X
C  T  A  B  L  E  C  T  W  K
```

# PARK

Find the words listed below in the square. If you want, check off the words as you find them.

## WORD LIST:

- ☐ TREES
- ☐ LAKE
- ☐ GRASS
- ☐ FLOWERS
- ☐ BENCH
- ☐ ANIMALS
- ☐ SLIDE
- ☐ FENCE
- ☐ SWING

| W | F | E | N | C | E | X | L | B | S |
|---|---|---|---|---|---|---|---|---|---|
| Z | L | L | P | Y | Y | O | A | E | U |
| F | L | O | W | E | R | S | K | N | G |
| S | F | E | N | X | V | I | E | C | R |
| W | C | Z | T | C | U | W | L | H | A |
| I | Z | P | E | S | L | I | D | E | S |
| N | A | N | I | M | A | L | S | F | S |
| G | R | T | R | E | E | S | X | W | N |

# ART

Find the words listed below in the square. If you want, check off the words as you find them.

## WORD LIST:

☐ COLOR     ☐ DRAW     ☐ CRAFT

☐ PAPER     ☐ PAINT     ☐ SEW

☐ CUT     ☐ GLUE     ☐ TAPE

```
L N C U T O K C C B
Q P A I N T D R O P
D D Q S M U T A L A
D Q H P W J M F O P
R G D C P L C T R E
A G L U E Z E F R R
W B V G H S E W K F
T A P E G E H B K I
```

# INSECTS

Find the words listed below in the square. If you want, check off the words as you find them.

## WORD LIST:

- ☐ ANT
- ☐ MOTH
- ☐ WASP
- ☐ EARWIG
- ☐ LADYBUG
- ☐ FLY
- ☐ CRICKET
- ☐ MOSQUITO
- ☐ BEE

| M | O | S | Q | U | I | T | O | A | F |
|---|---|---|---|---|---|---|---|---|---|
| U | D | A | S | E | F | T | X | C | L |
| S | U | E | A | R | W | I | G | R | Y |
| B | N | G | K | R | V | D | I | I | L |
| T | P | B | T | E | Q | J | A | C | E |
| M | O | T | H | S | X | E | N | K | O |
| L | A | D | Y | B | U | G | T | E | A |
| J | W | A | S | P | B | E | E | T | F |

# TRAVEL

Find the words listed below in the square. If you want, check off the words as you find them.

## WORD LIST:

☐ CAR     ☐ BUS     ☐ BOAT

☐ TRAIN     ☐ SUBWAY     ☐ TRUCK

☐ PLANE     ☐ VAN     ☐ BIKE

```
P  B  I  K  E  E  T  B  M  T
L  V  R  J  Z  Q  G  W  B  R
A  V  T  R  A  I  N  O  O  U
N  Q  Q  V  B  L  N  E  A  C
E  N  U  X  B  U  S  Y  T  K
K  T  D  C  Z  A  F  S  J  U
S  U  B  W  A  Y  J  A  L  D
I  V  A  N  J  T  C  A  R  A
```

# COLORING PAGES

This section is full of coloring pages. The goal is to color in the pictures any way you would like!

## An Example

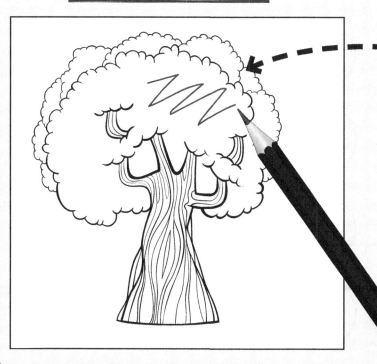

Take some time to color the picture.

Try out your pencil crayons or other coloring tools on the next page.

# HAVE FUN COLORING

You can use any combination of colors, on the following pages, that make you smile!

# A QUOTATION OR SAYING ON THE BACK OF EACH PAGE

On the back each coloring page is a delightful quotation in light gray. We did this so that nothing on the back of your coloring page will effect your lovely work of art.

# TRY OUT YOUR COLORS

Sometimes it can be nice to test out some of the colors that you are planning to use on the coloring pages. You can do that in the circles below:

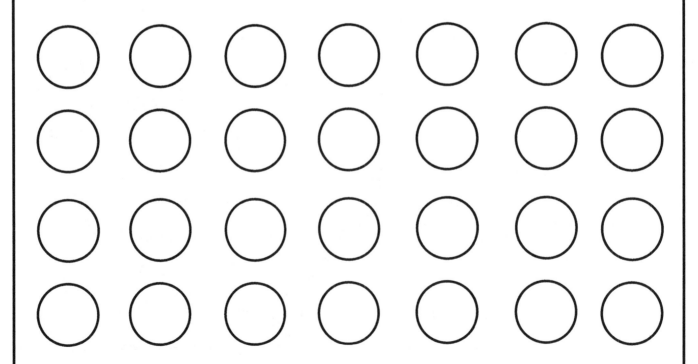

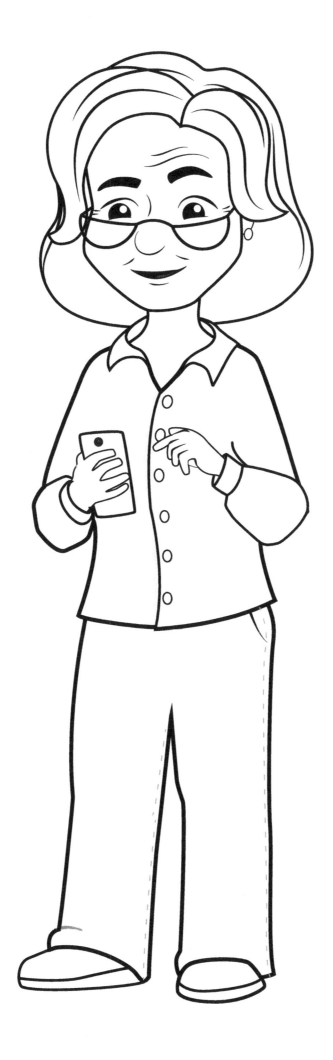

# "A warm smile is the universal language of kindness."

– William Arthur Ward

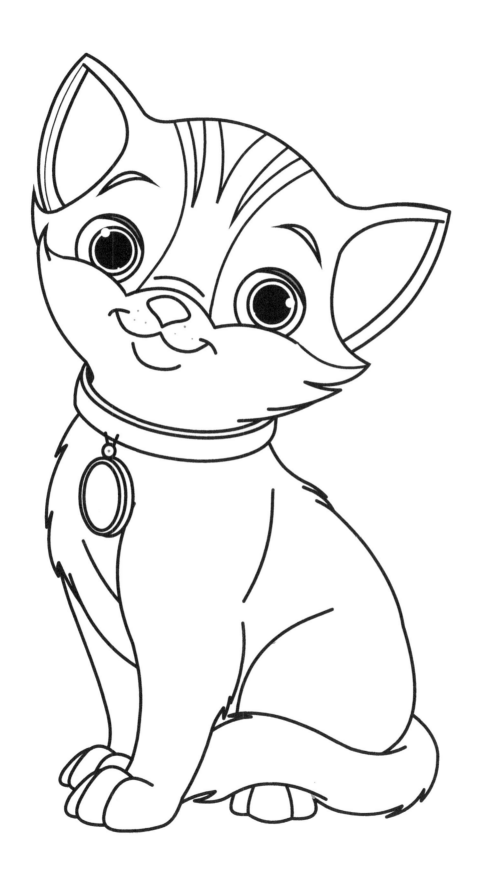

**" I am beginning to learn it is the sweet, simple things of life which are the real ones after all. "**

– Laura Ingalls Wilder

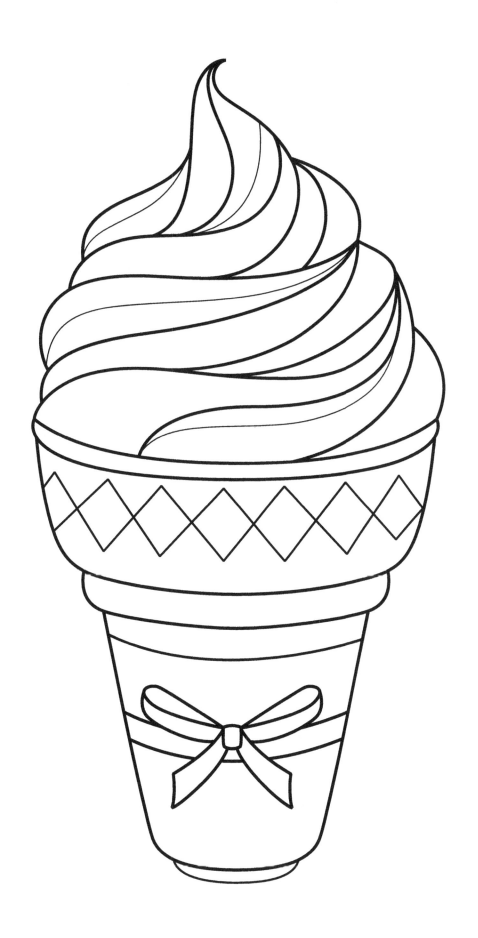

# "Well done is better than well said.

– Benjamin Franklin

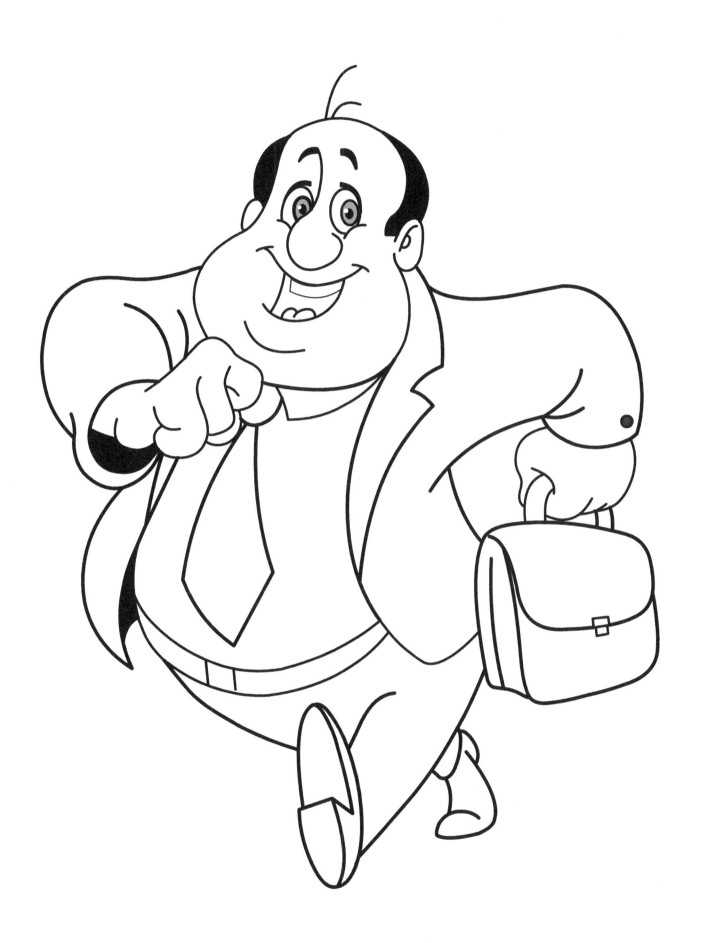

# "The earth laughs in flowers."

– Ralph Waldo Emerson

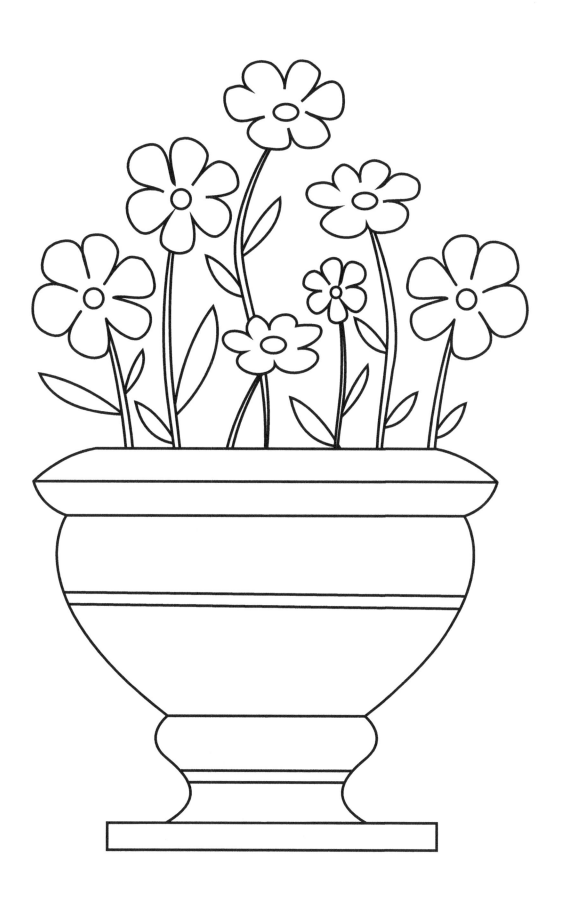

# "When one door of happiness closes, another opens.

– Helen Keller

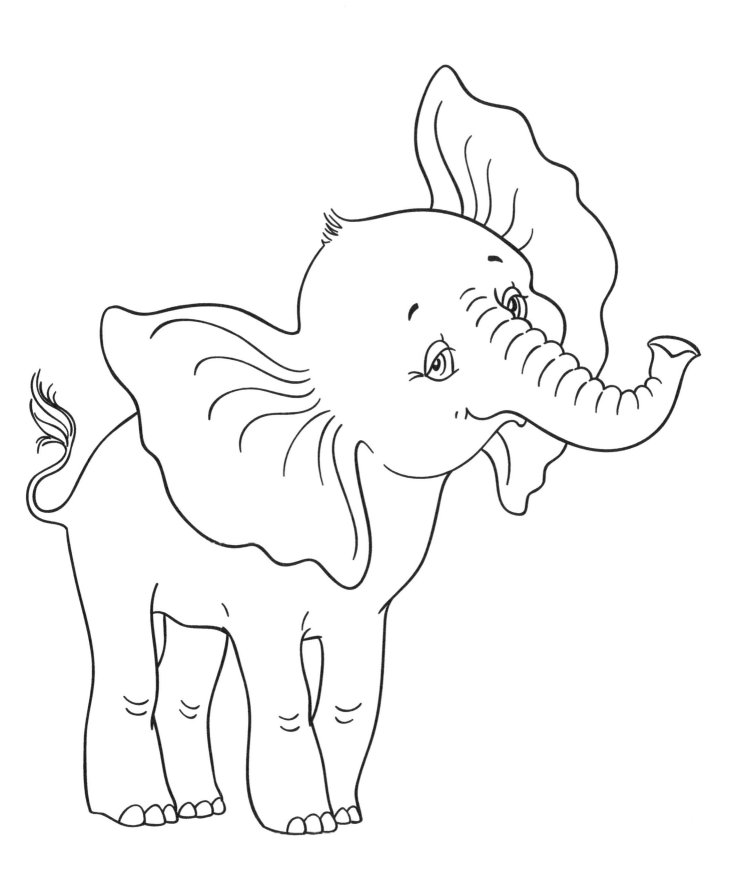

# "Each day bring its own gifts.

– Marcus Aurelius

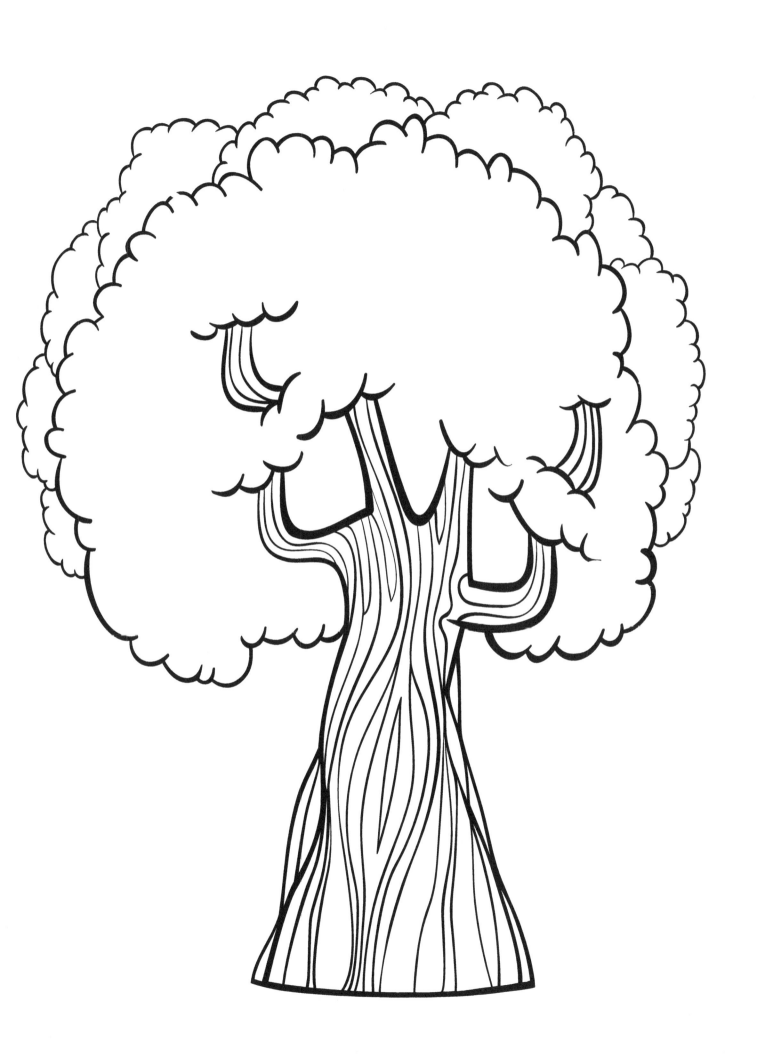

# "Wisdom begins in wonder.

– Socrates

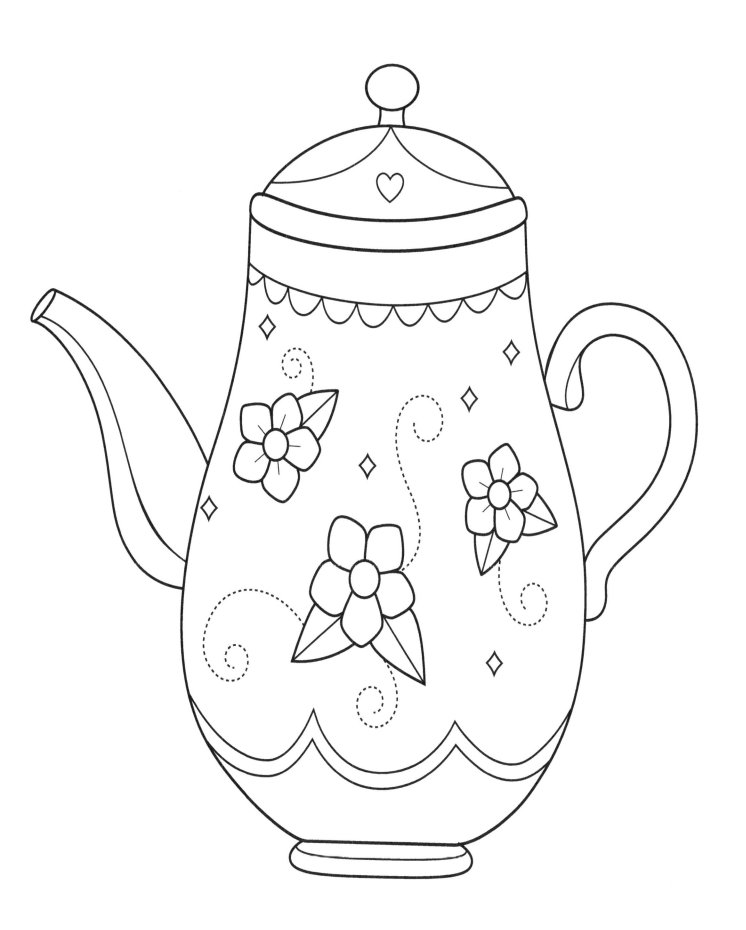

# "Be yourself, everyone else is already taken."

– Oscar Wilde

# FIND THE DIFFERENCES

This section is full of 'Find the Differences' puzzles. The goal is to find three differences between the pictures.

## An Example

Find the 3 Differences Between the Trumpets

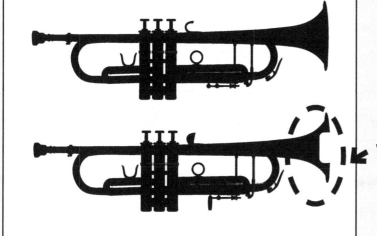

HINT: Each puzzle has 3 differences.

This area of the trumpet is different from the other trumpet.

# FIND 3 DIFFERENCES BETWEEN THE MEN STUDYING PLANS

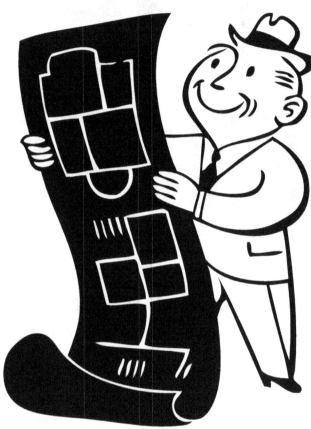

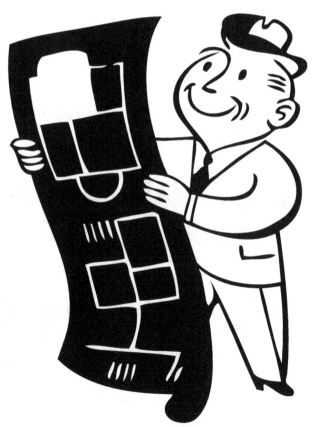

# FIND 3 DIFFERENCES
# BETWEEN THE SET OF CARDS

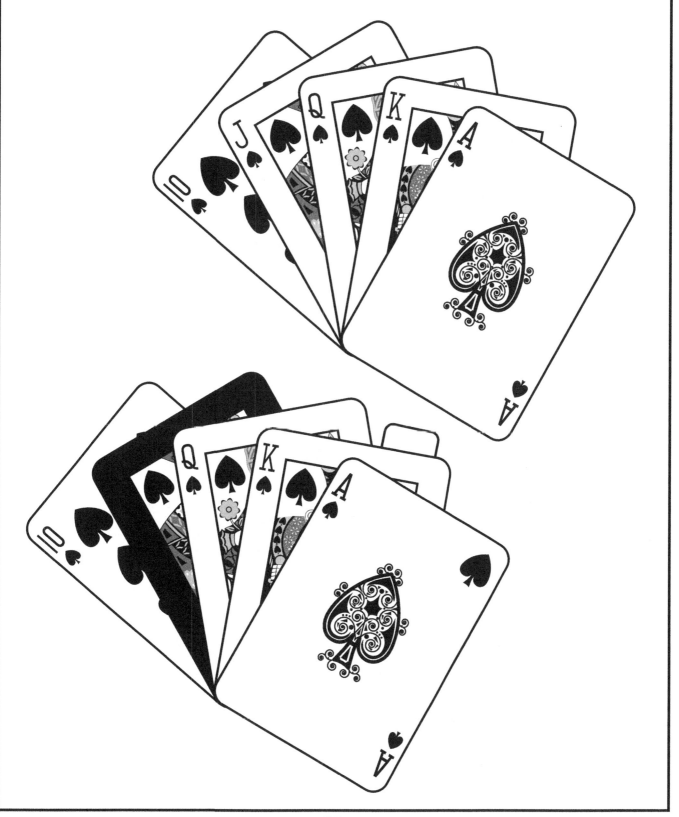

# FIND 3 DIFFERENCES
# BETWEEN THE RADIO PLAYERS

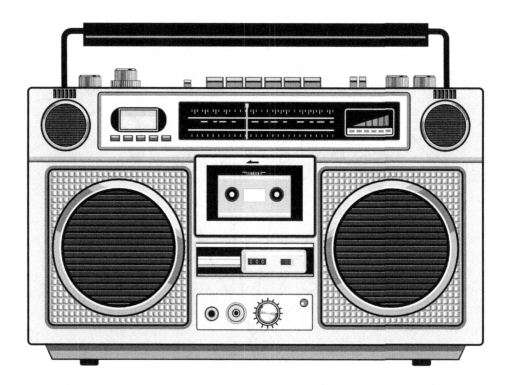

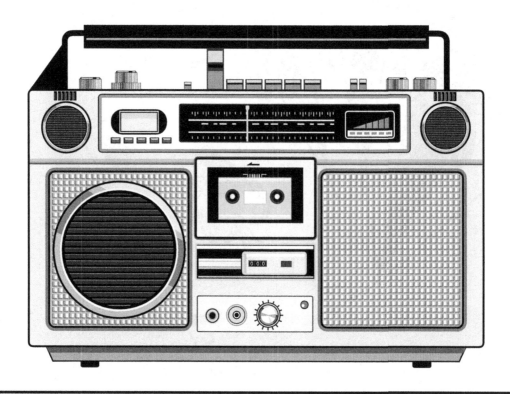

# FIND 3 DIFFERENCES
# BETWEEN THE DANCERS

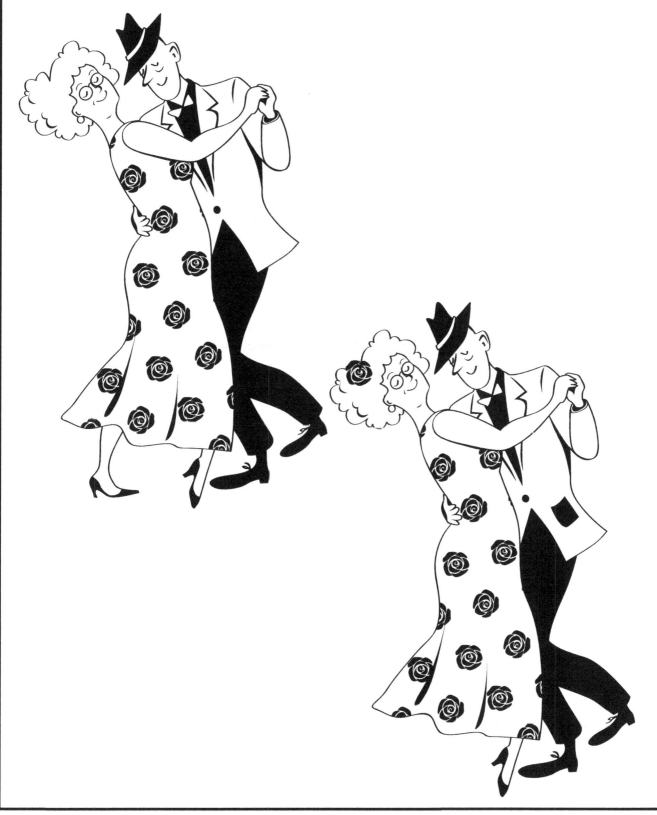

# FIND 3 DIFFERENCES BETWEEN THE LIVING ROOM SCENES

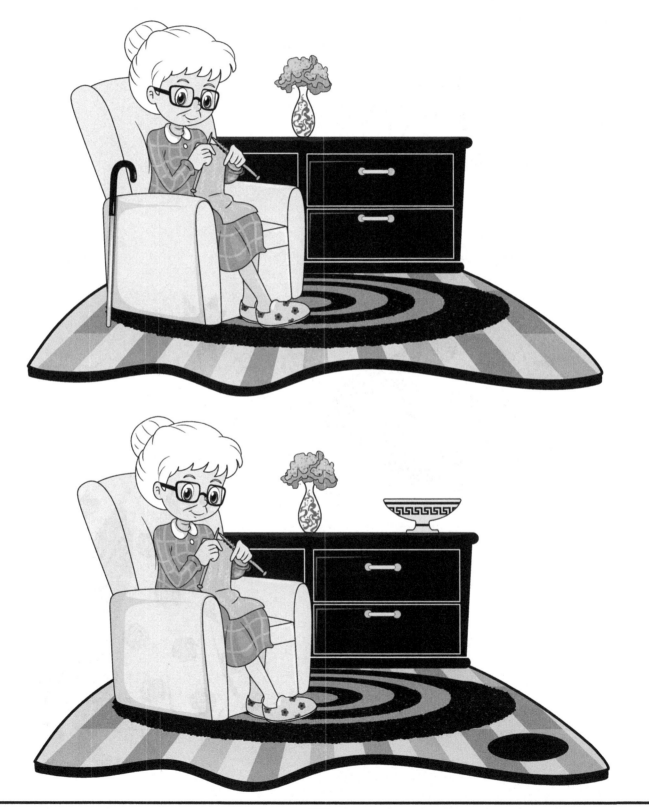

# FIND 3 DIFFERENCES
# BETWEEN THE CLASSIC CARS

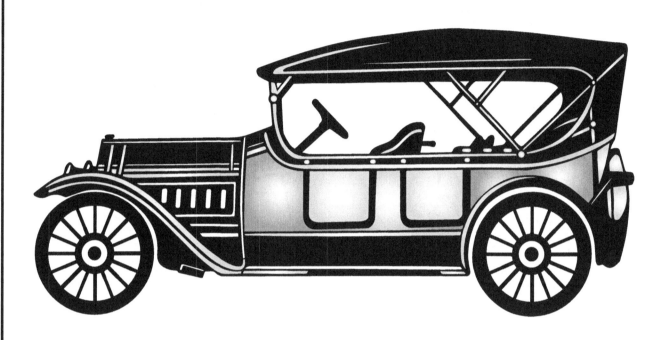

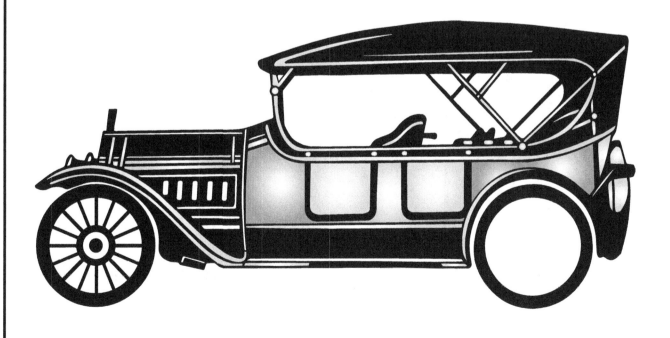

# FIND 3 DIFFERENCES
# BETWEEN THE DOCTORS

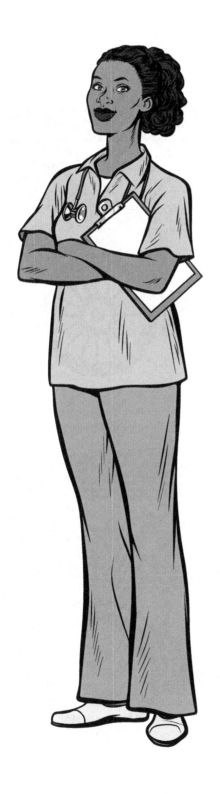
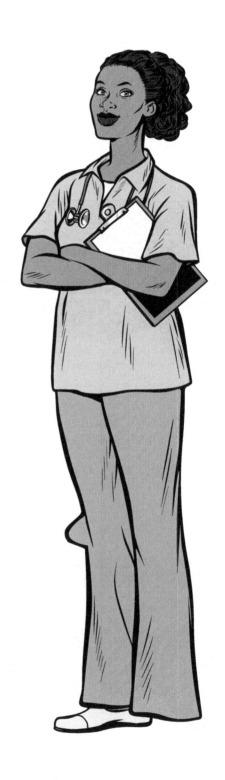

# FIND 3 DIFFERENCES BETWEEN THE TRAYS OF CUPCAKES

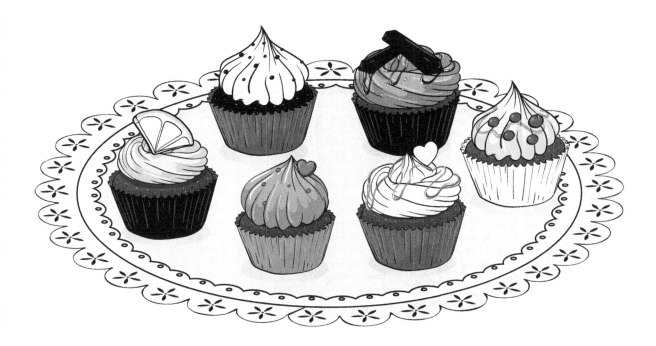

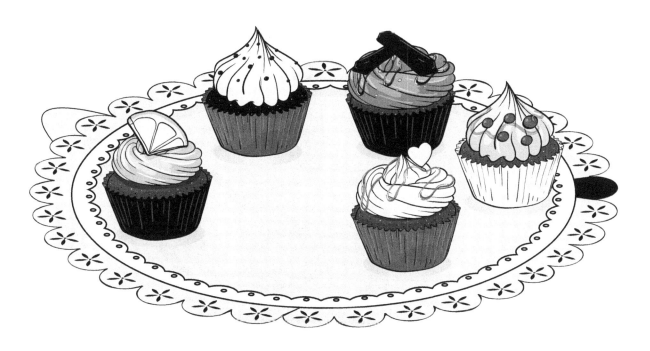

# FIND 3 DIFFERENCES BETWEEN THE FARMERS ON TRACTORS

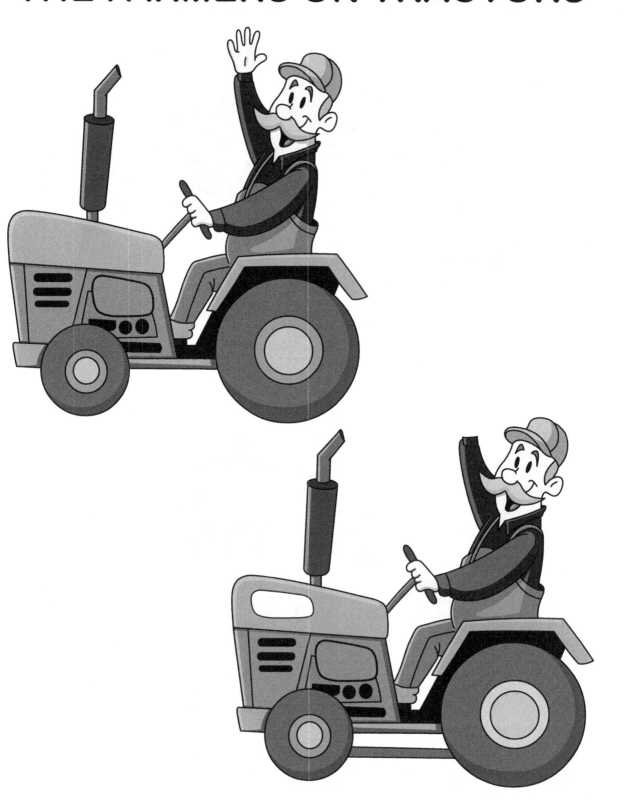

# FIND 3 DIFFERENCES
# BETWEEN THE HAPPY PIGS

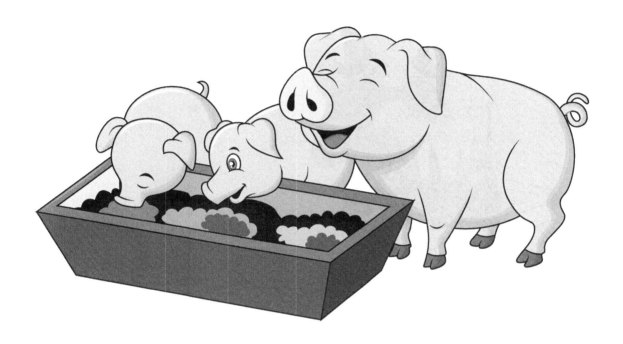

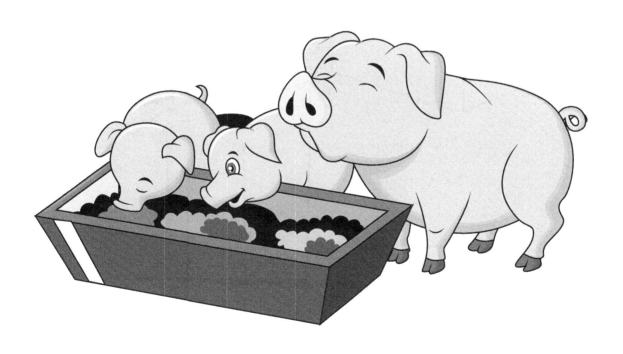

# FIND 3 DIFFERENCES BETWEEN THE LADIES DOING LAUNDRY

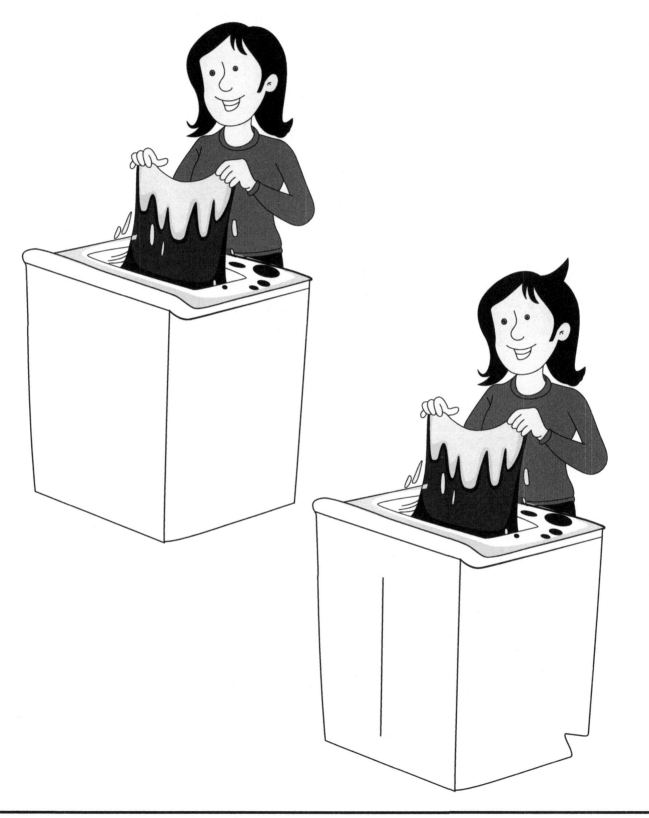

# FIND 3 DIFFERENCES
# BETWEEN THE SIDE TABLES

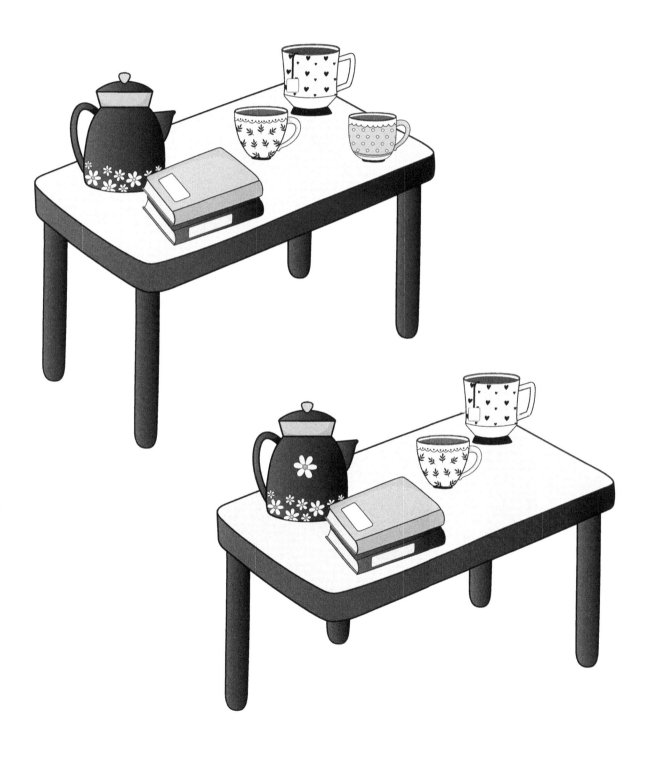

# FIND 3 DIFFERENCES
# BETWEEN THE BUSINESS MEN

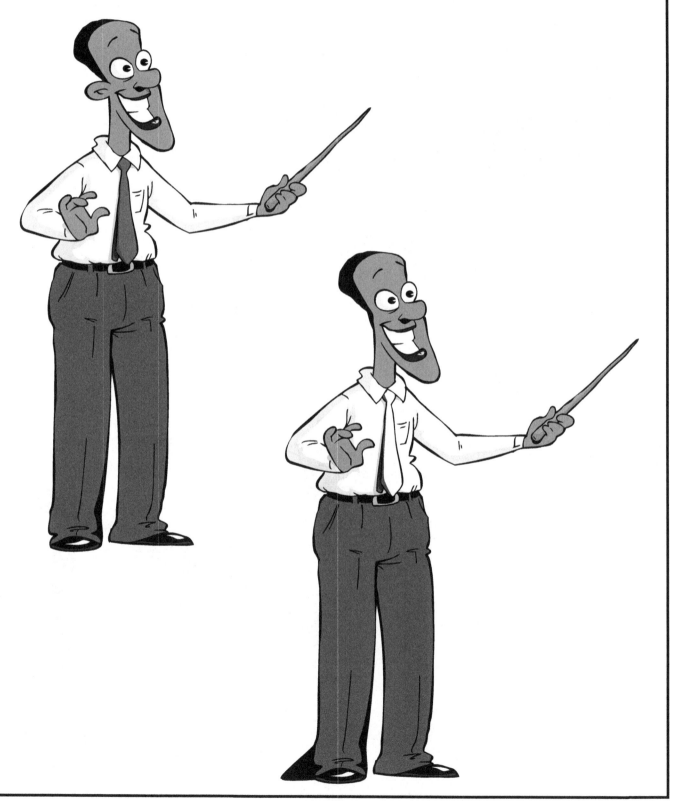

# SPOT THE STARS

This section is full of 'Spot the Stars' puzzles. The goal is to find five stars in each picture.

## An Example

Spot the 5 Stars that are Hidden in the Picture Below

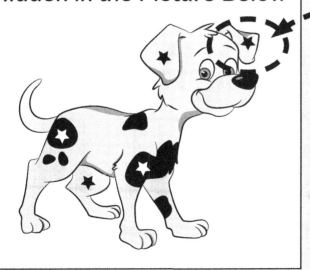

Here is one of the hidden stars in this picture.

Hint: Each puzzle has 5 hidden stars.

# SPOT THE 5 STARS WHICH
# ARE HIDDEN IN THE SIGN

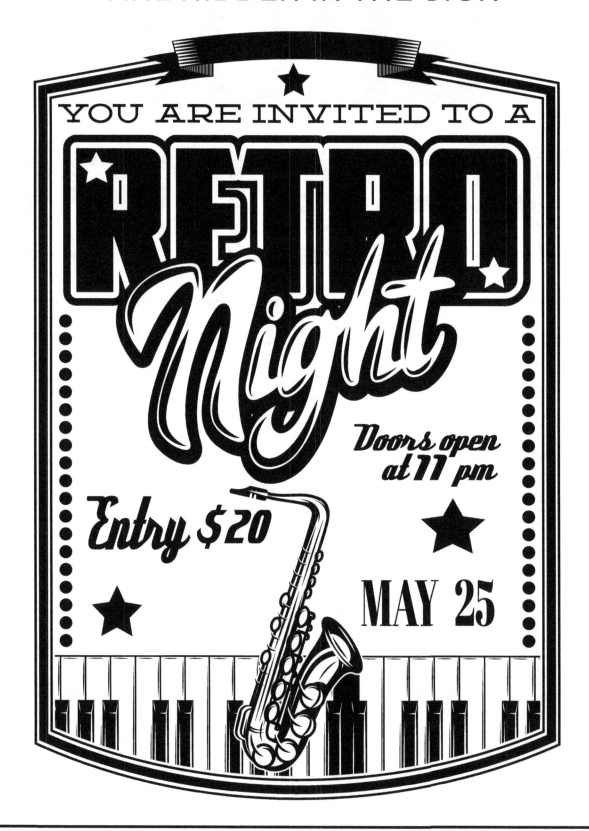

# SPOT THE 5 STARS WHICH ARE
# HIDDEN IN THE DINING SCENE

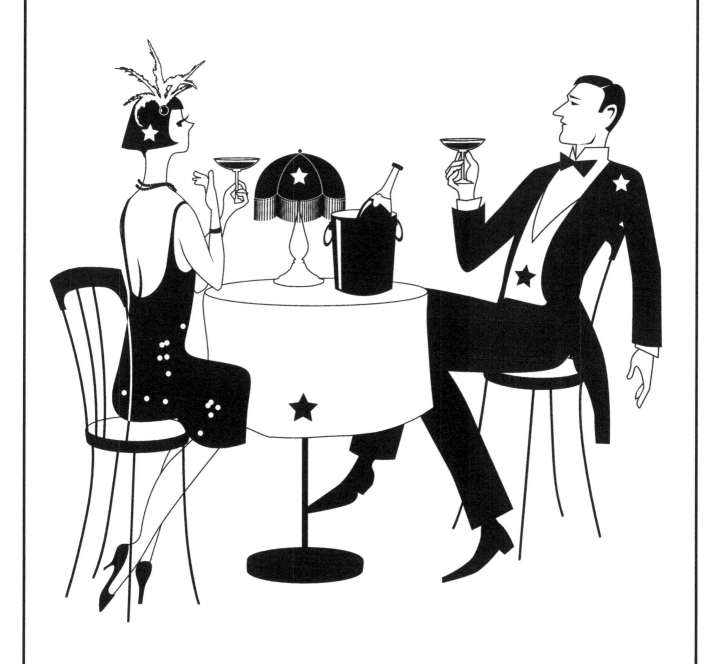

# SPOT THE 5 STARS WHICH ARE HIDDEN IN THE GARDENING SCENE

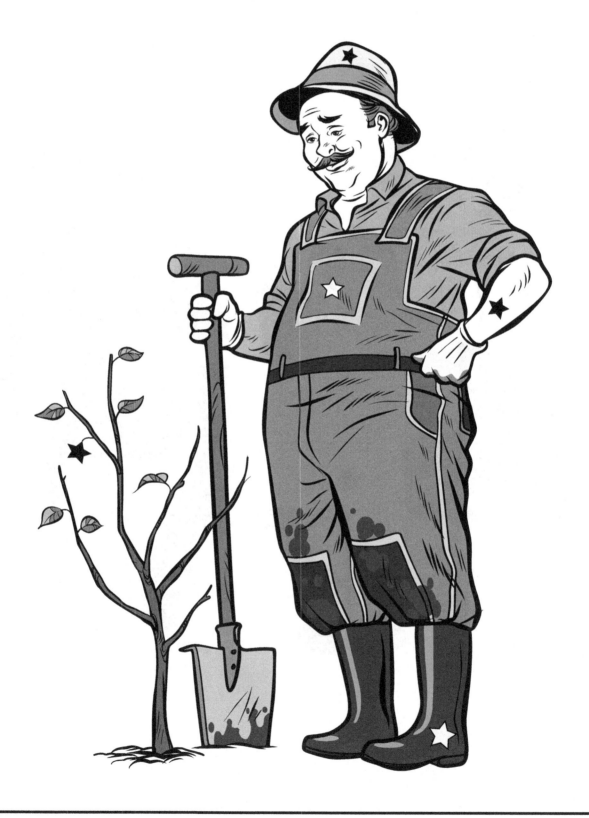

# SPOT THE 5 STARS WHICH ARE
# HIDDEN IN THE DOG WALKING SCENE

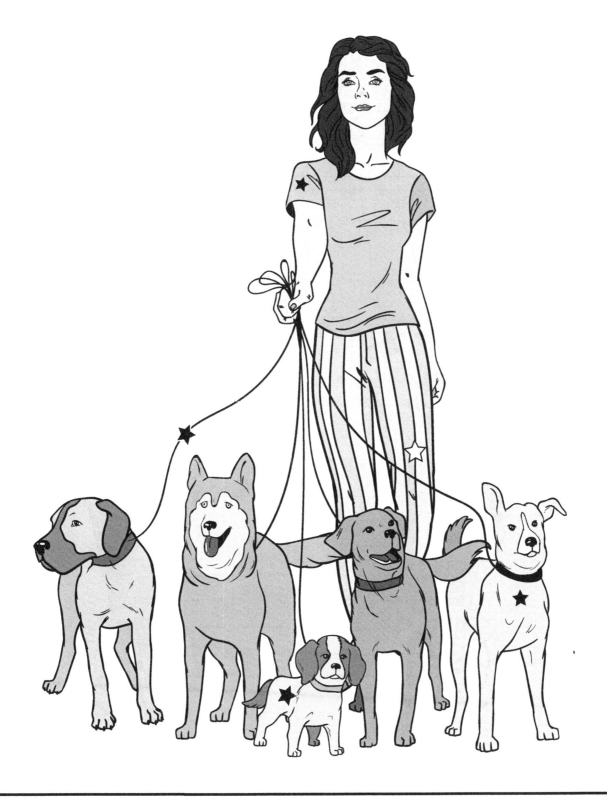

# SPOT THE 5 STARS WHICH ARE HIDDEN IN THE FLOWER CART

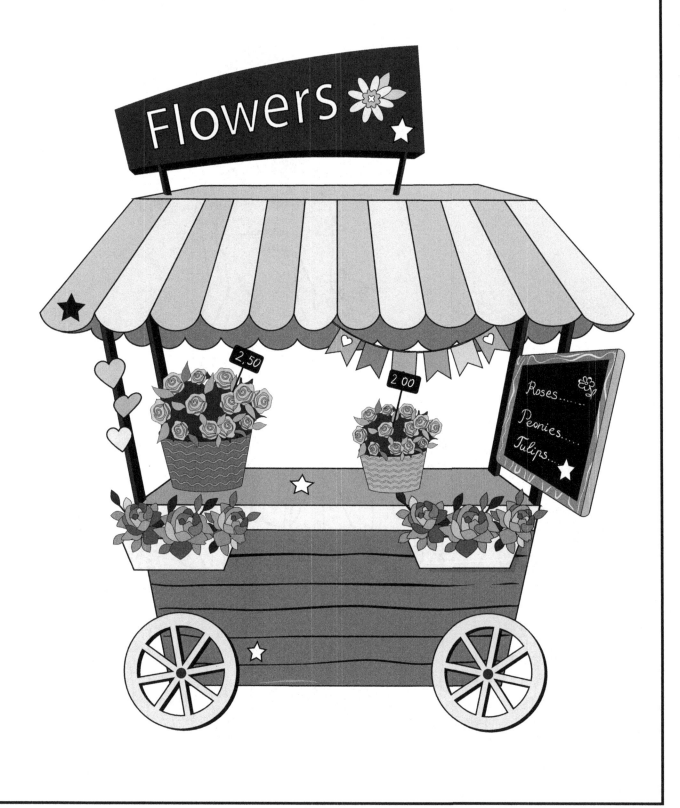

# SPOT THE 5 STARS WHICH ARE HIDDEN IN THE LUGGAGE TROLLEY

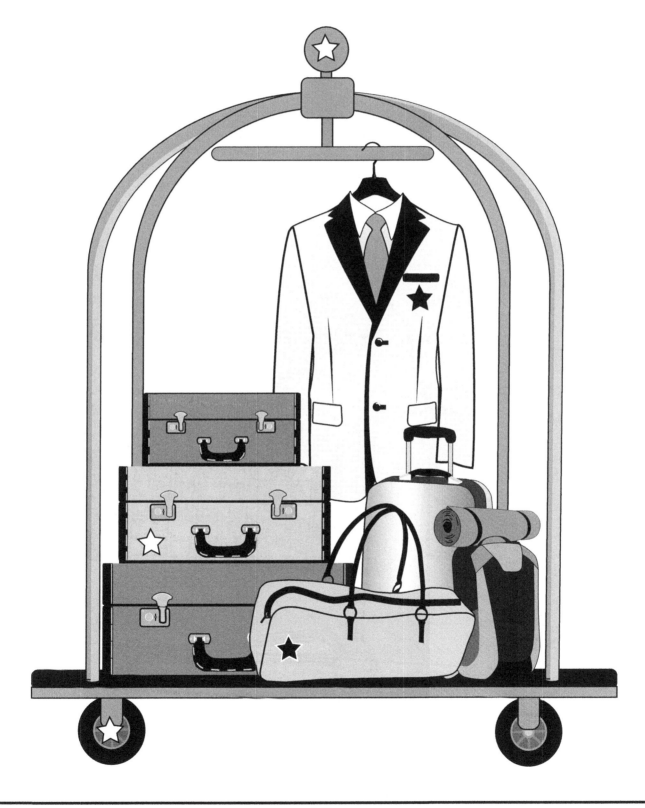

# SPOT THE 5 STARS WHICH ARE HIDDEN IN THE SHOPPING SCENE

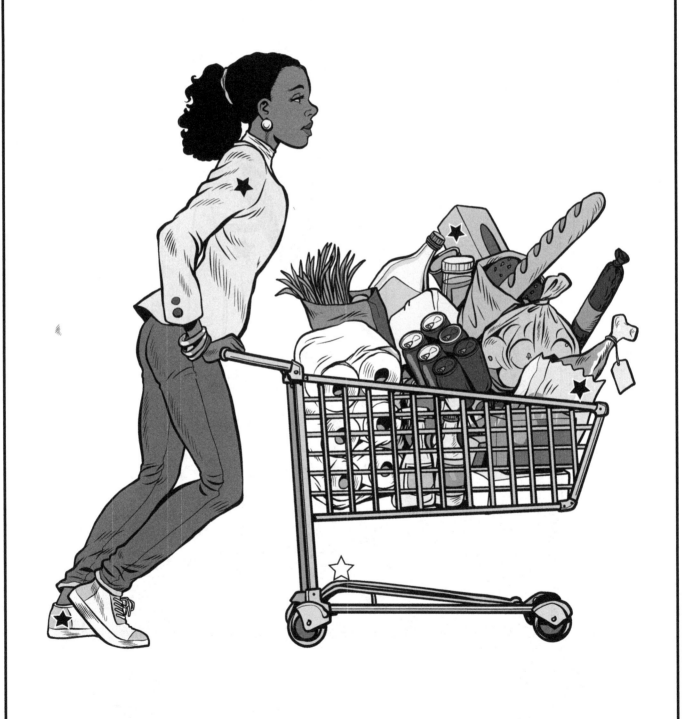

# SPOT THE 5 STARS WHICH ARE HIDDEN IN THE BIKING SCENE

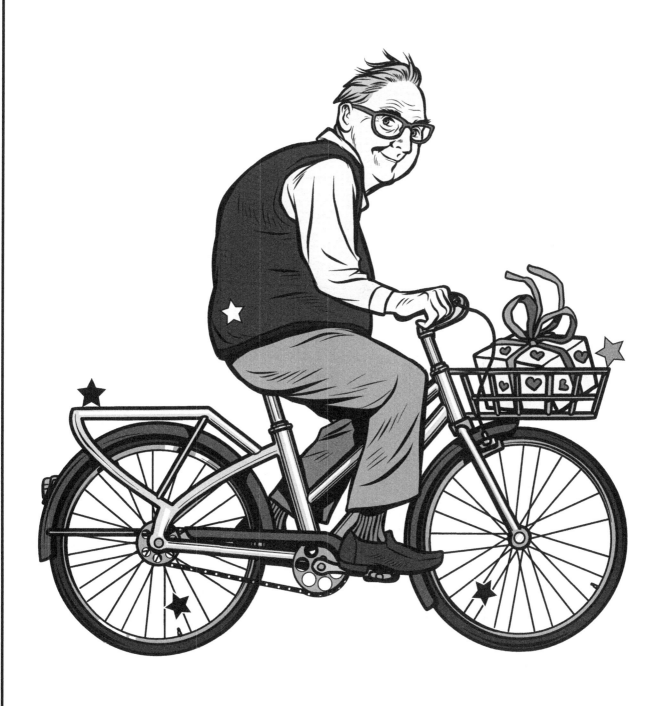

# SPOT THE 5 STARS WHICH ARE HIDDEN IN THE ISLAND SCENE

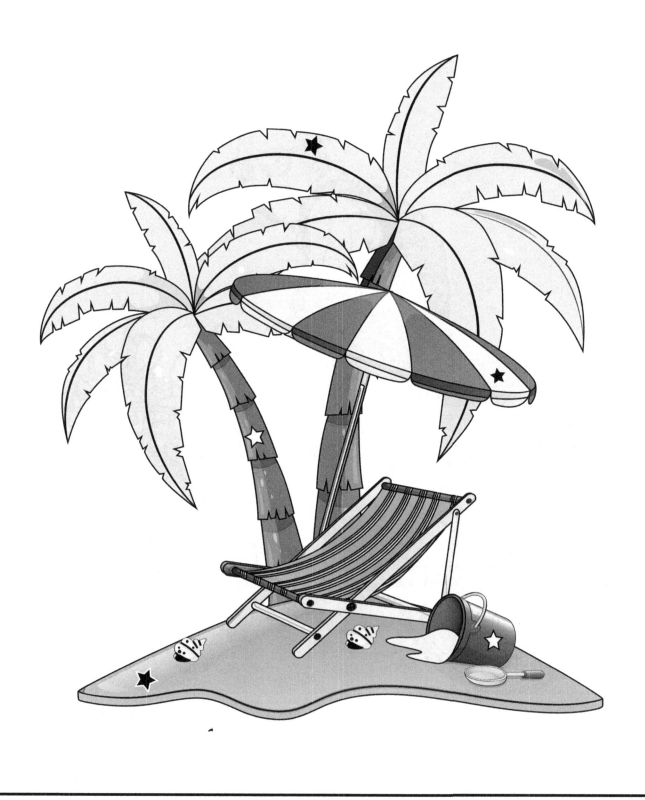

# SPOT THE 5 STARS WHICH ARE HIDDEN IN THE BIRD HOUSE SCENE

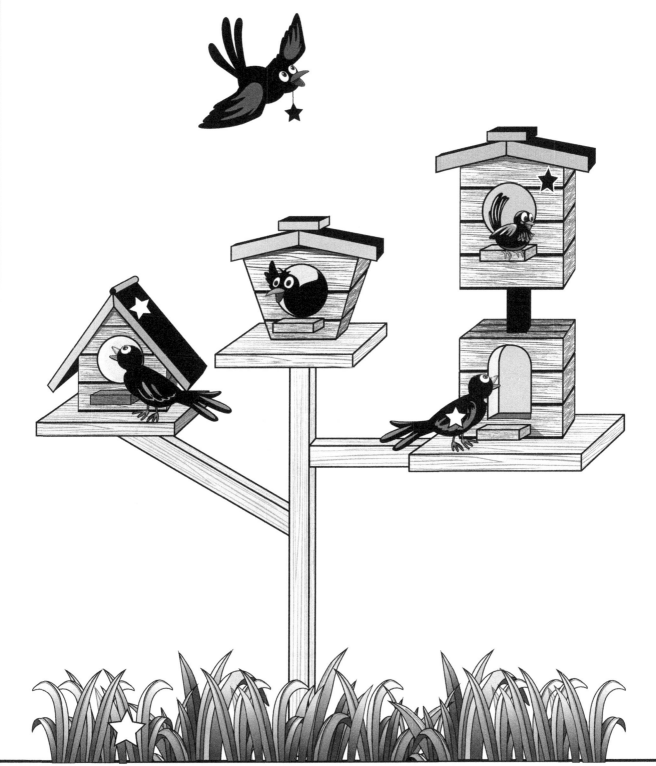

# SPOT THE FIVE STARS WHICH ARE HIDDEN IN THE DELIVERY SCENE

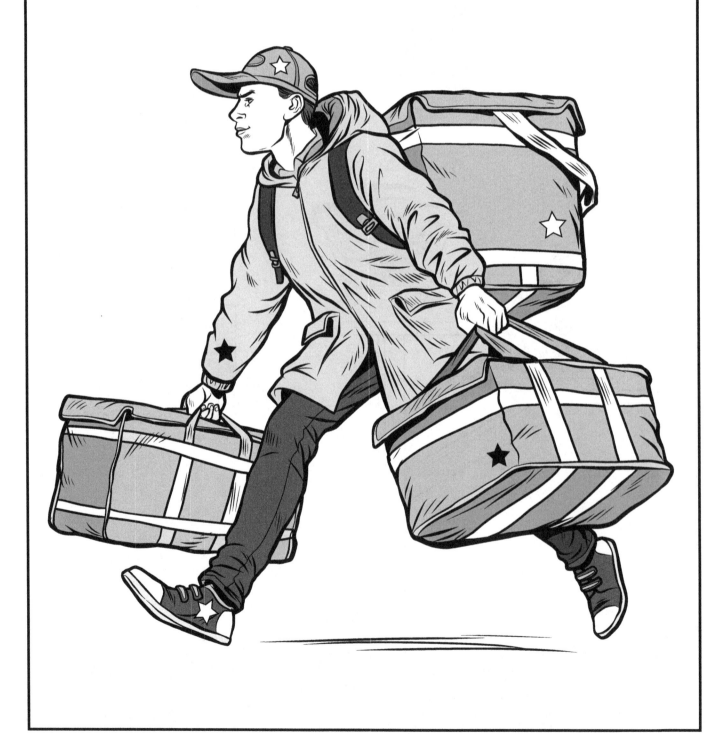

# MAZES

This section is full of mazes. The goal for each maze is to draw a line that goes from start to finish.

## An Example

Draw a Line that Takes You From Start to Finish

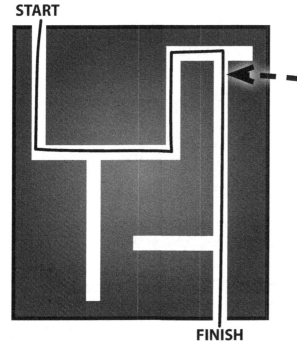

START

FINISH

Here is the path that goes from the start of the maze to the end of the maze.

# DRAW A LINE THAT TAKES YOU
# FROM START TO FINISH

START

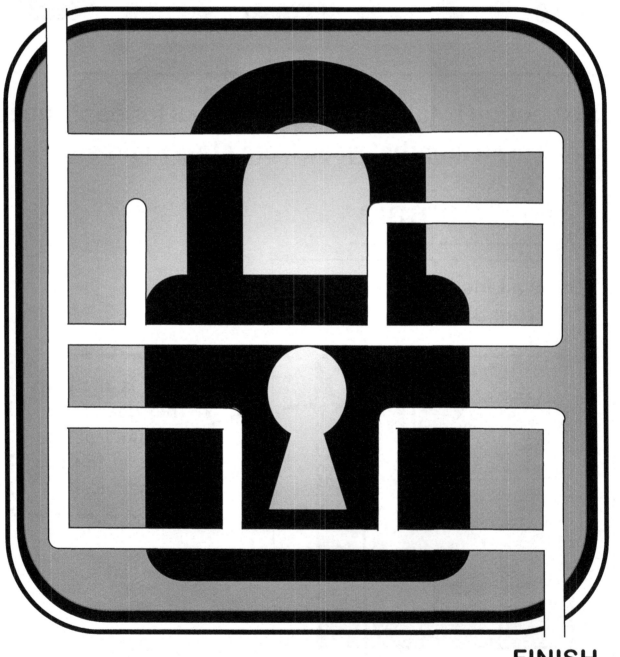

FINISH

# DRAW A LINE THAT TAKES YOU
# FROM START TO FINISH

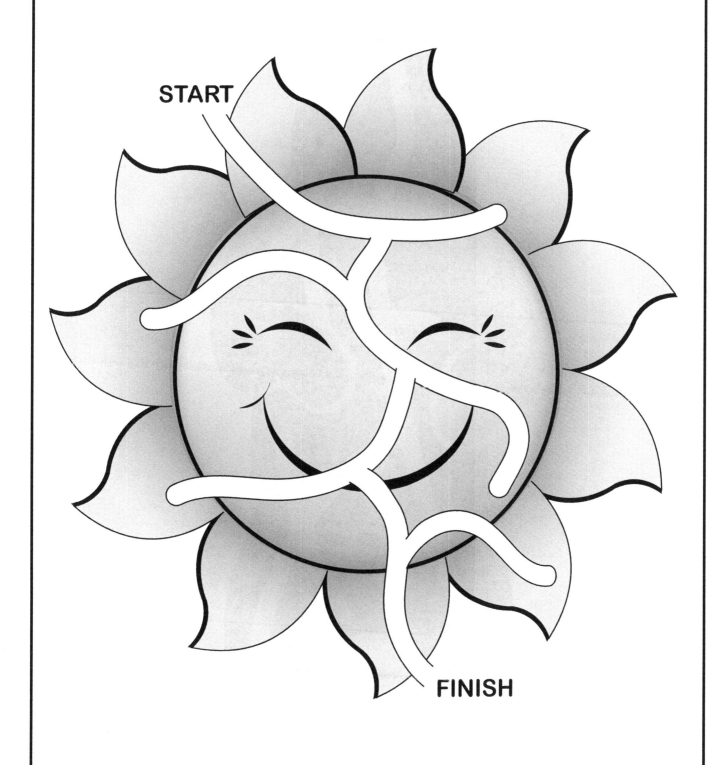

# DRAW A LINE THAT TAKES YOU
# FROM START TO FINISH

START

FINISH

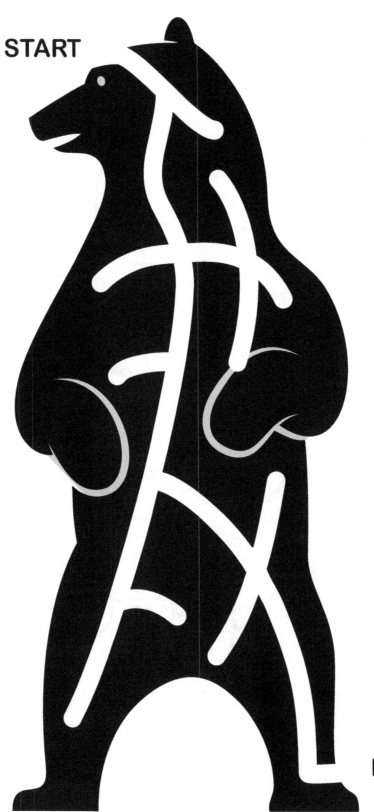

# DRAW A LINE THAT TAKES YOU
# FROM START TO FINISH

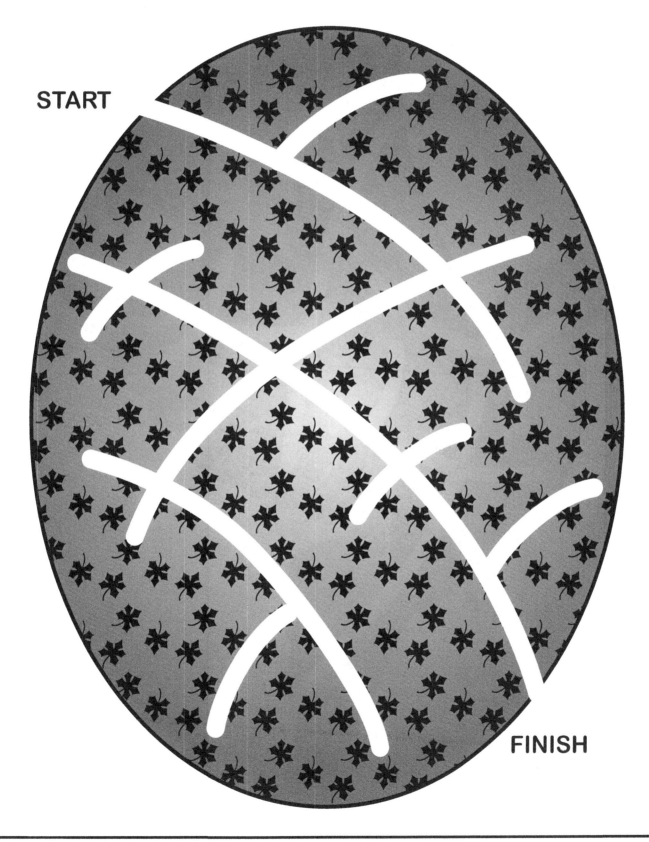

START

FINISH

# DRAW A LINE THAT TAKES YOU
# FROM START TO FINISH

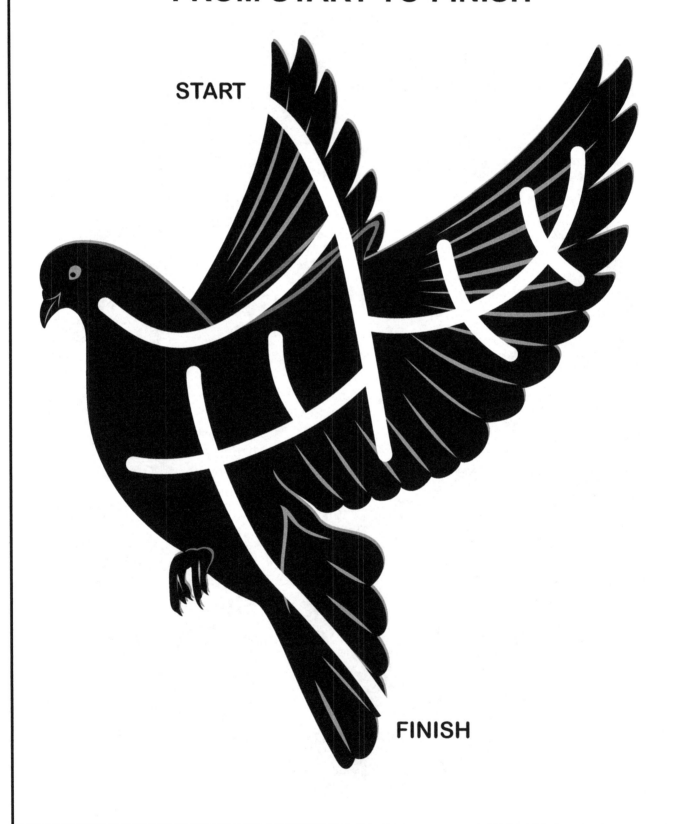

START

FINISH

# DRAW A LINE THAT TAKES YOU
# FROM START TO FINISH

**START**

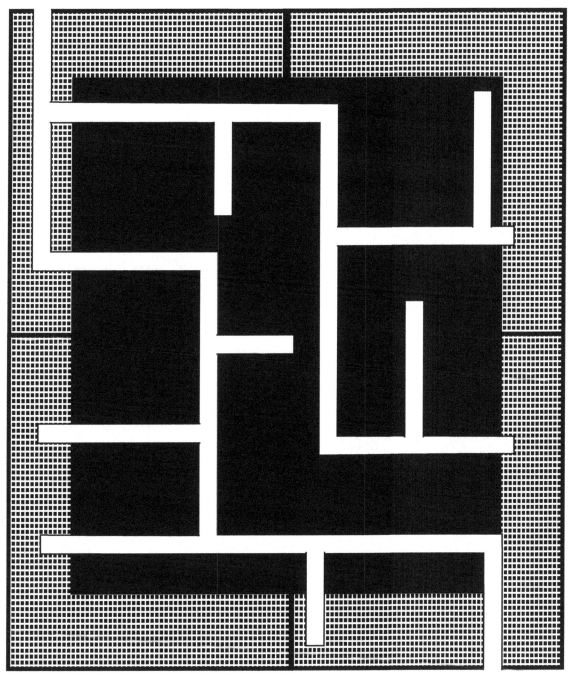

**FINISH**

# DRAW A LINE THAT TAKES YOU
# FROM START TO FINISH

START

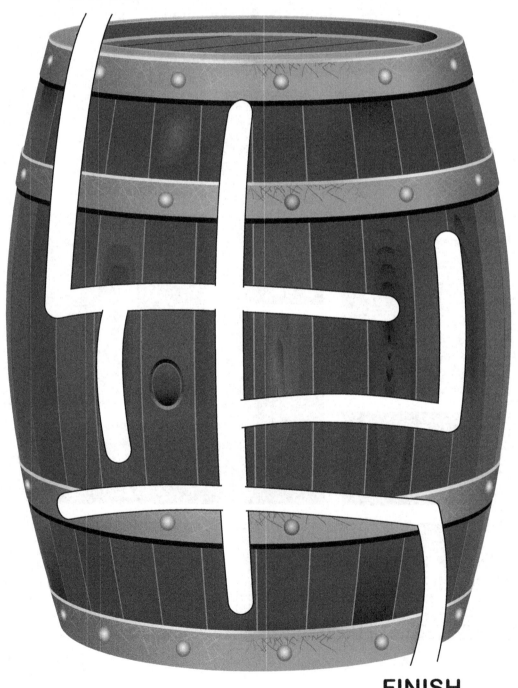

FINISH

# DRAW A LINE THAT TAKES YOU
# FROM START TO FINISH

START

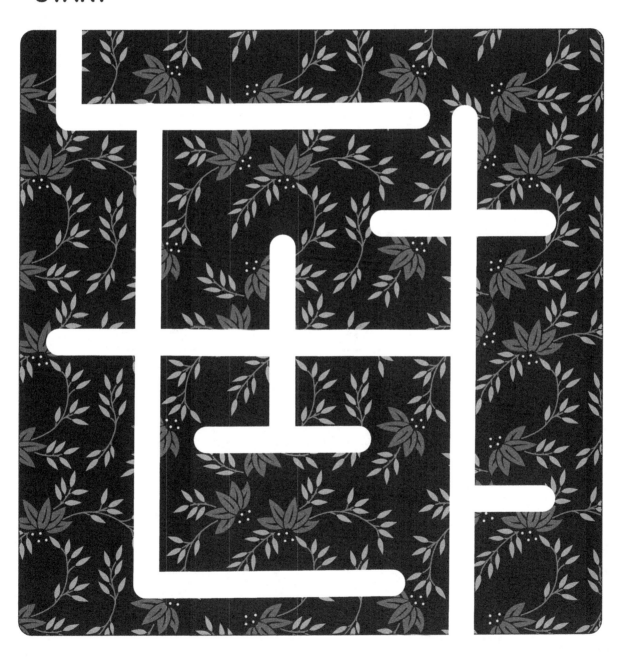

FINISH

# DRAW A LINE THAT TAKES YOU
# FROM START TO FINISH

START

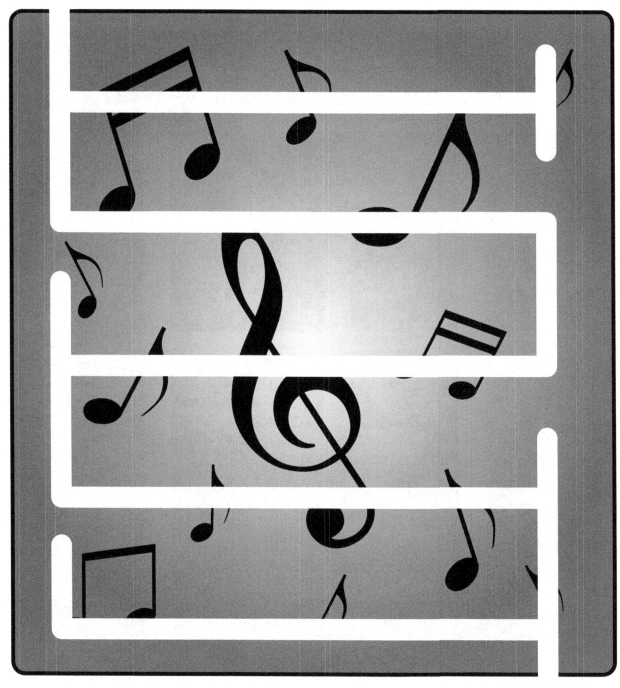

FINISH

# DRAW A LINE THAT TAKES YOU
# FROM START TO FINISH

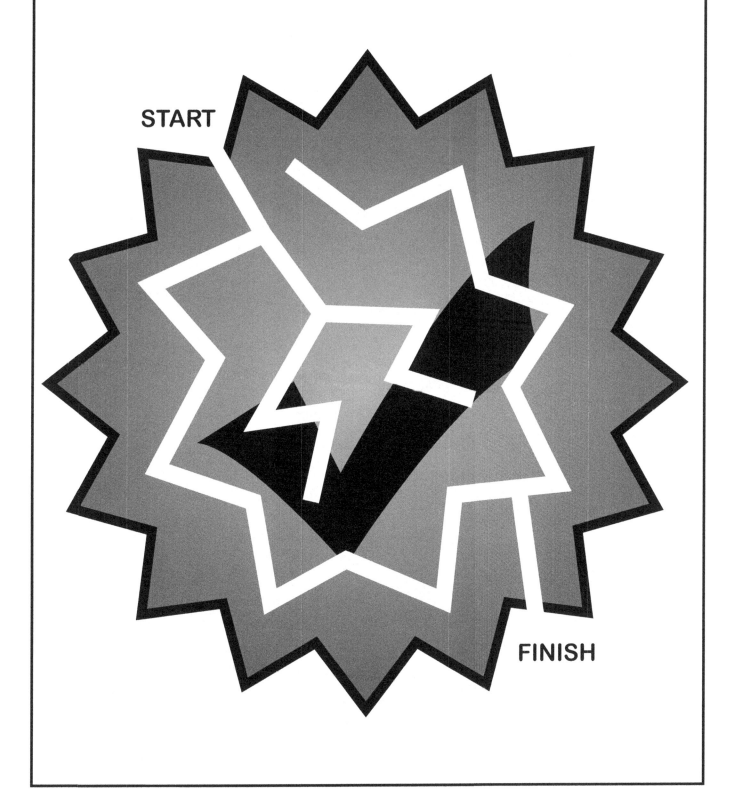

START

FINISH

# DRAW A LINE THAT TAKES YOU
# FROM START TO FINISH

START

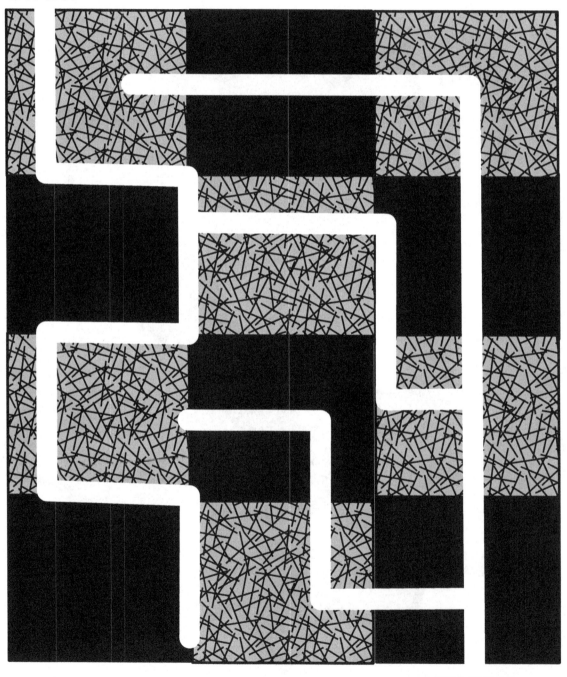

FINISH

# DRAW A LINE THAT TAKES YOU
# FROM START TO FINISH

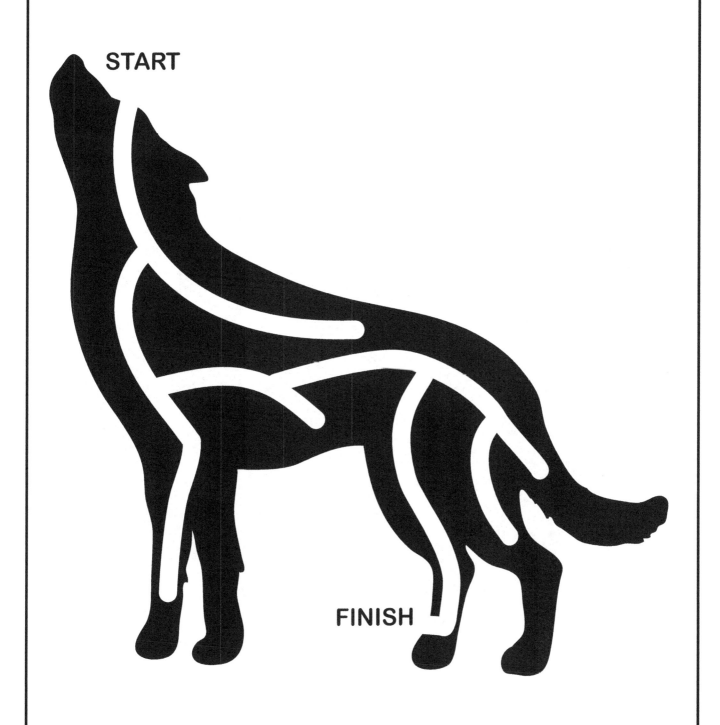

# DRAW A LINE THAT TAKES YOU
# FROM START TO FINISH

START

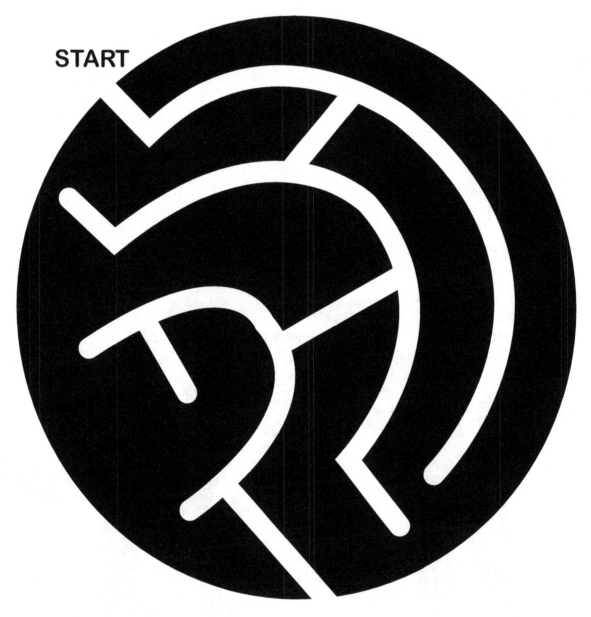

FINISH

# THE ANSWERS

This section has the answers for each puzzle. Each puzzle is identified by its page number.

## An Example

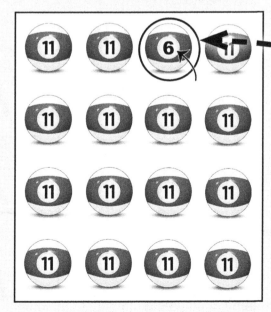

Page 20

The answer to the puzzle is circled.

The answer section is ordered by page number.

Page
6

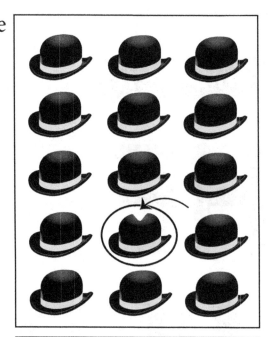

Page
7

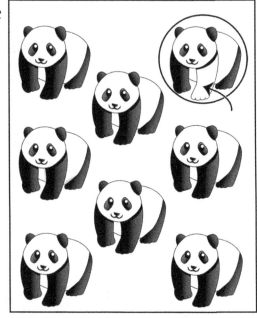

Page
8

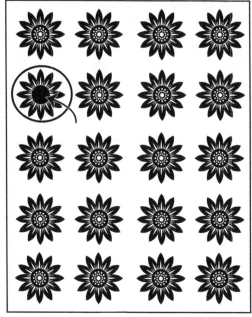

Page
9

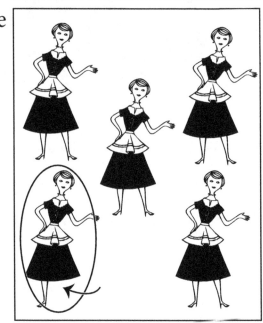

Page
10

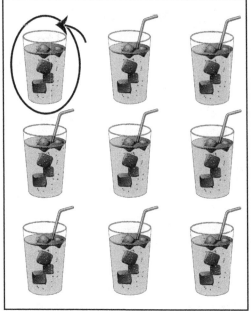

Page
11

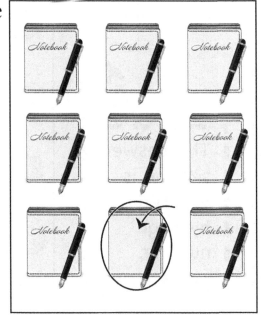

Page
12

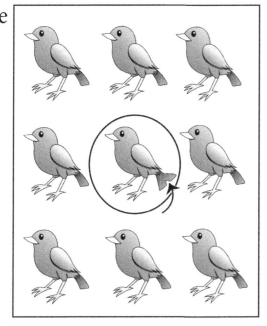

Page
13

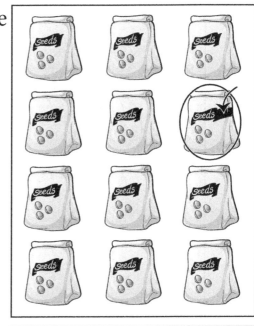

Page
14

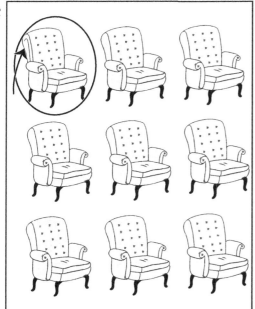

Page
15

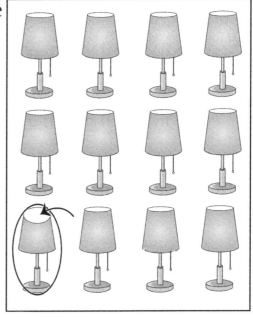

Page
16

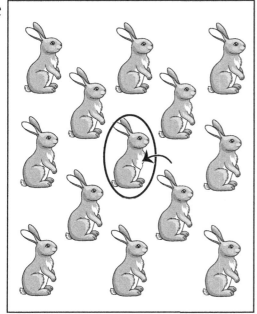

Page
17

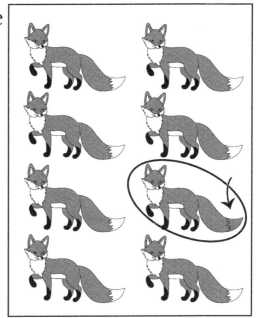

Page 18

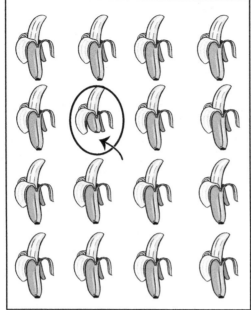

Page 19

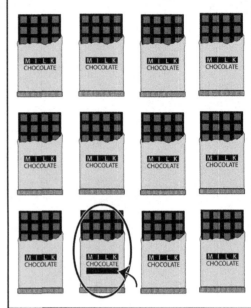

Page 20

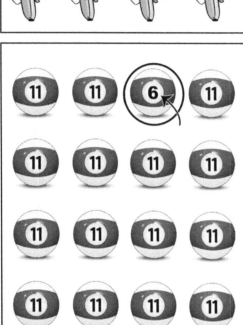

END OF
SPOT THE ODD ONE
OUT SOLUTIONS

***

START OF WORD
SEARCHES
SOLUTIONS

Page 22: Radio

Page 23: Farm

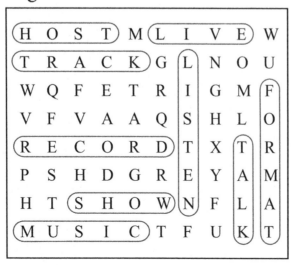

## Page 24: Cards

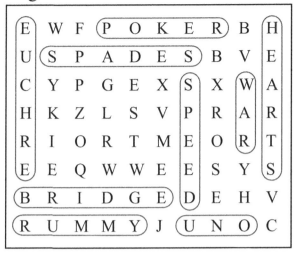

## Page 25: Happy

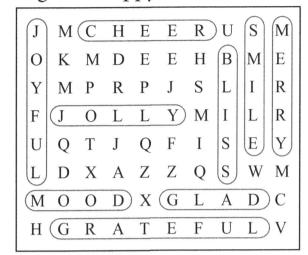

## Page 26: Vegetables

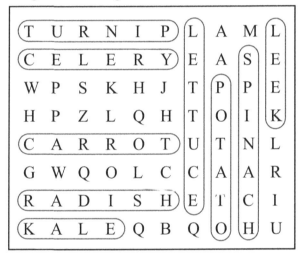

## Page 27: That's Funny

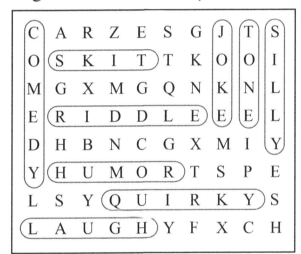

## Page 28: Bedroom

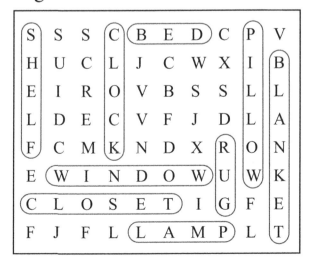

## Page 29: Telephone

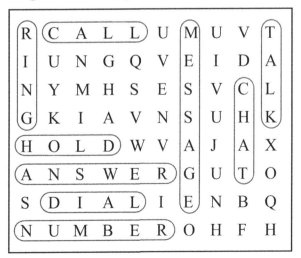

## Page 30: Haircut

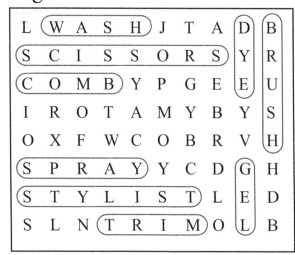

## Page 31: Pets

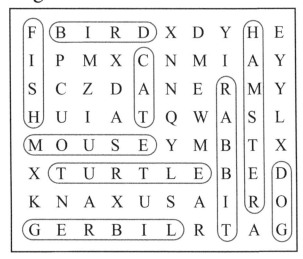

## Page 32: Kitchen

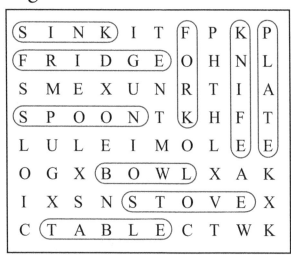

## Page 33: Park

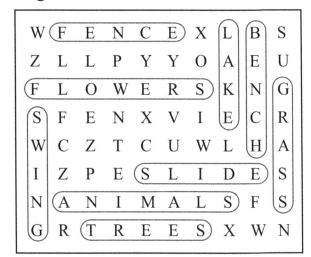

## Page 34: Art

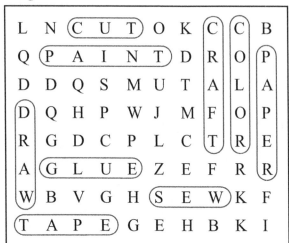

## Page 35: Insects

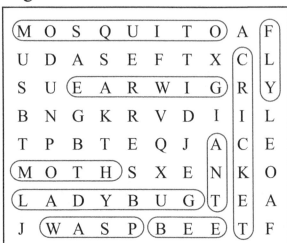

## Page 36: Travel

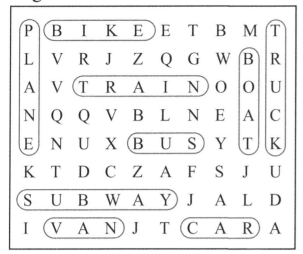

END OF WORD
SEARCH SOLUTIONS

***

START OF FIND THE
DIFFERENCE SOLUTIONS

## Page 56: Man with Plans

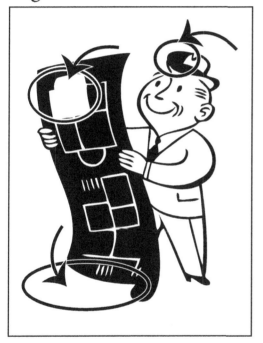

## Page 57: Cards

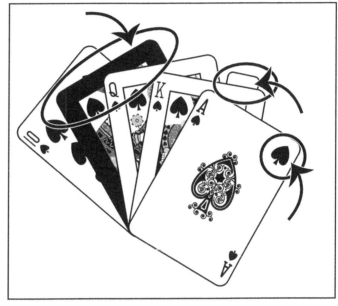

## Page 59: Dancers

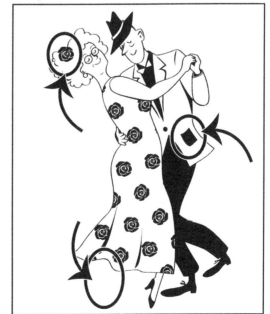

## Page 58: Radio

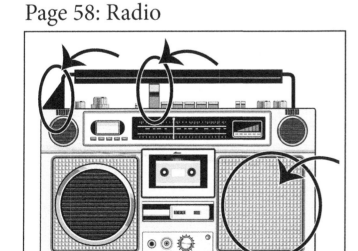

## Page 60: Lady in Living Room

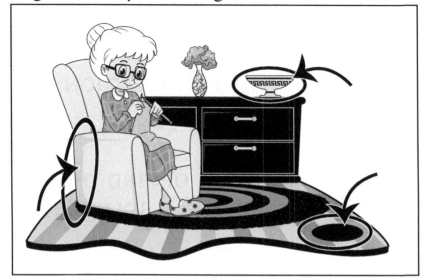

## Page 62: Doctor

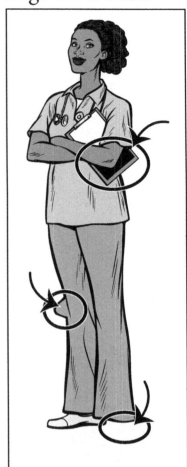

## Page 61: Classic Car

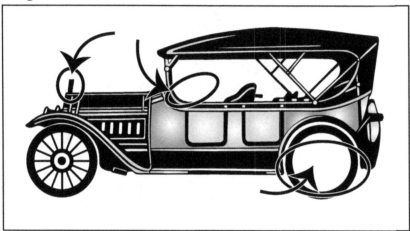

## Page 63: Cupcake Tray

## Page 64: Farmer on a Tractor

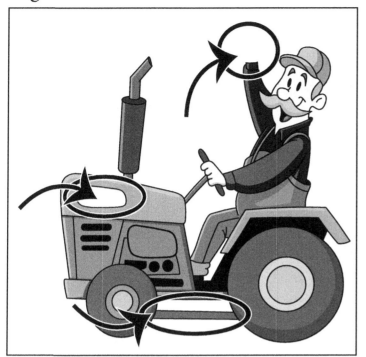

## Page 65: Happy Pigs

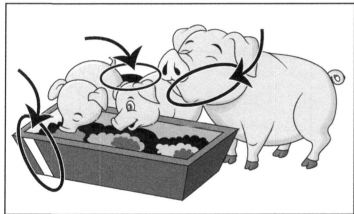

## Page 67: Table

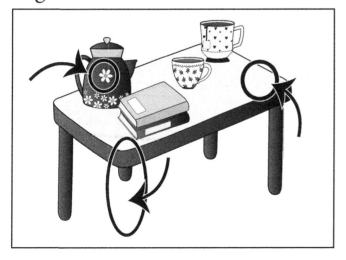

## Page 66: Laundry

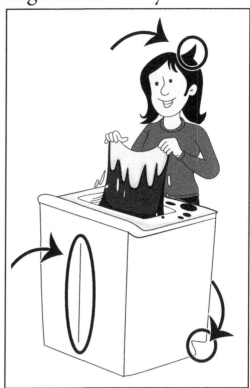

## Page 68: Business Man

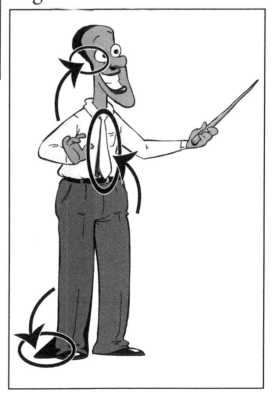

Page 70

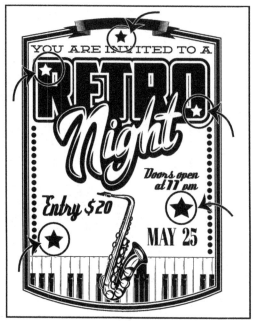

Page 71

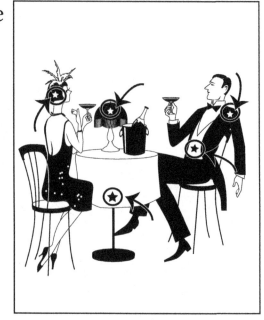

Page 72

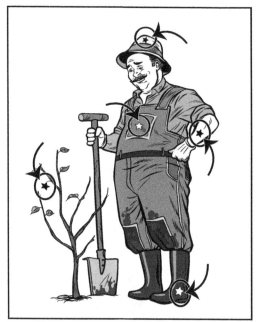

Page 73

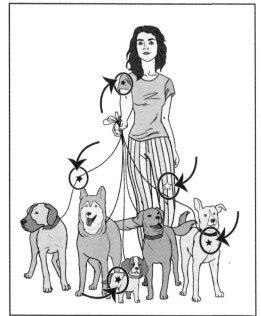

Page 74

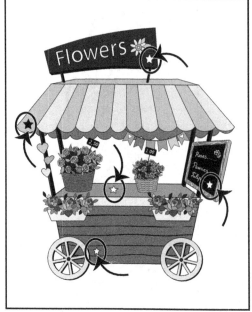

Page 75

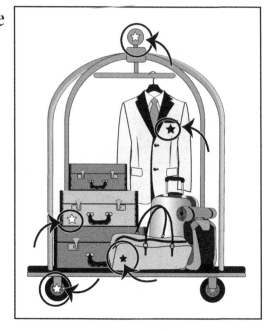

Page
76

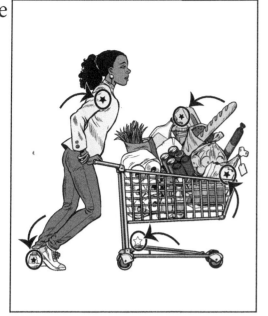

Page
77

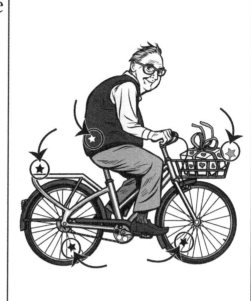

Page
78

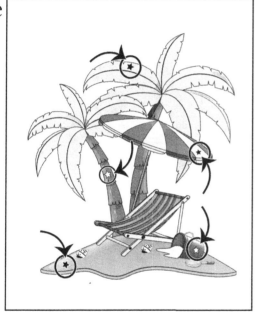

Page
79

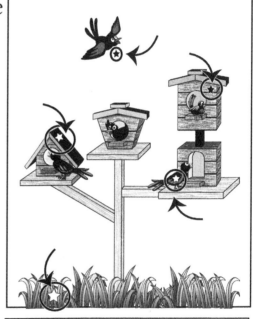

Page
80

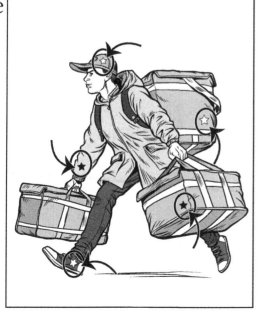

**END OF
FIND THE STARS
SOLUTIONS**

**✳✳✳**

**START OF MAZE
SOLUTIONS**

Page
82

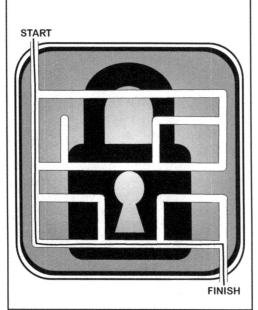

Page
83

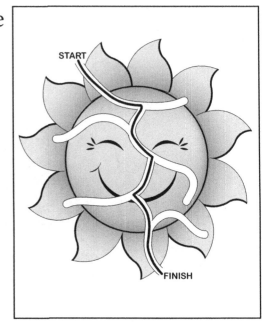

Page
84

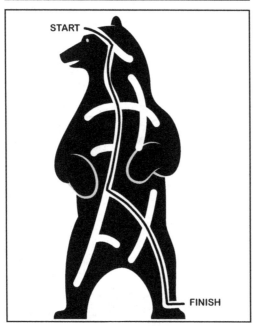

Page
85

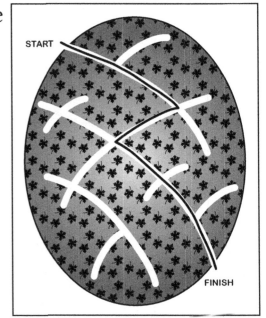

Page
86

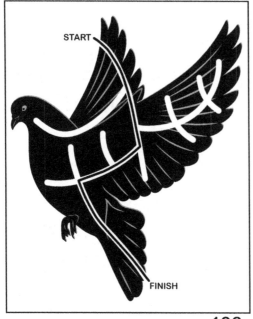

Page
87

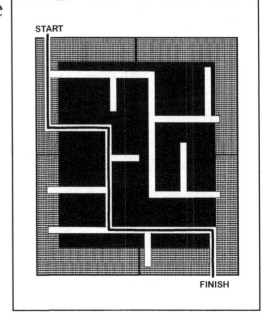

Page
88

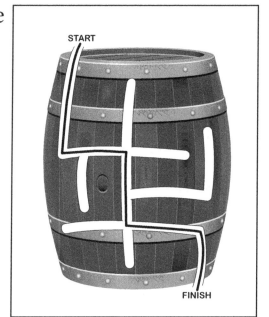

Page
89

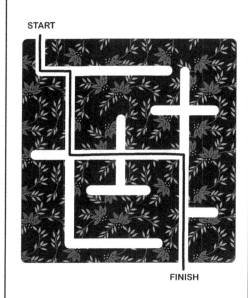

Page
90

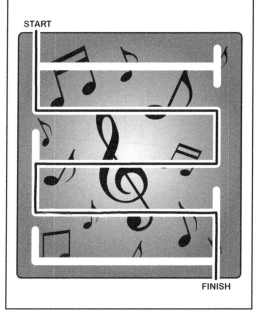

Page
91

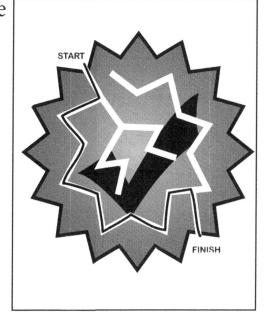

Page
92

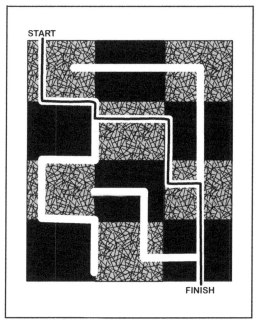

Page
93

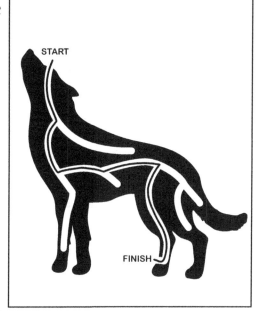

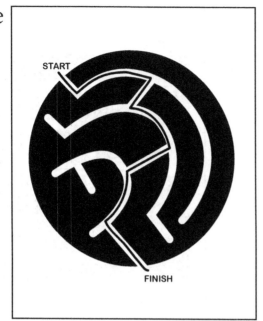

START

FINISH

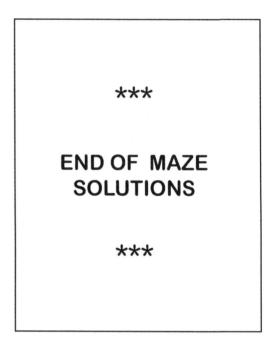

***

END OF MAZE
SOLUTIONS

***

## For more books like this one consider:

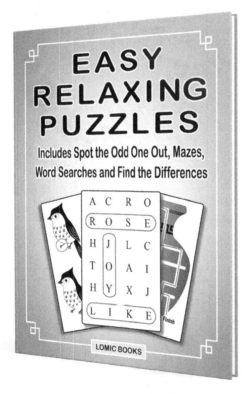

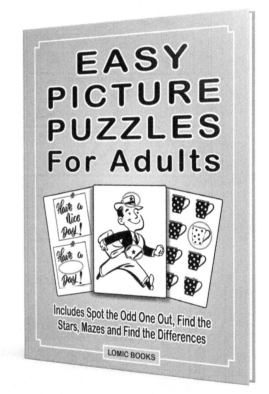

Both books are the same level as this book, and offer lots of fun activities.

For more information check out:

www.lomicbooks.com

Thank you!

Made in the USA
Coppell, TX
01 July 2021